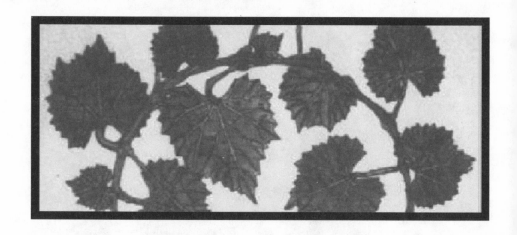

Muscadine

Medicine

Diane K. Hartle, Ph.D.

Phillip Greenspan, Ph.D.

James L. Hargrove, Ph.D.

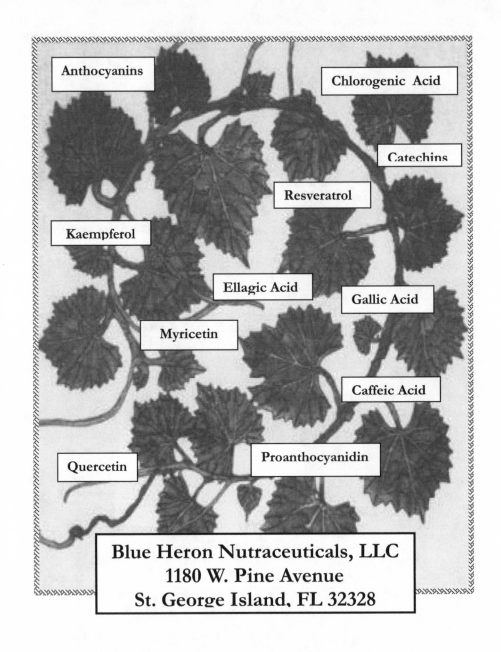

Blue Heron Nutraceuticals, LLC
1180 W. Pine Avenue
St. George Island, FL 32328

ISBN Number 1-4116-4397-6

First Edition

Muscadine Medicine

Chapters

Acknowledgments

We thank the men, women and families who make their livings growing muscadine grapes and producing specialty products from this very special American vine. You are a daily inspiration to us. We thank the many scientists who have discussed their current research with us, and the efforts of the farmers' and growers' associations devoted to informing more people about the health benefits of muscadine and scuppernong grapes.

~Caveats~

Chapter 1 – Introducing Muscadines and Muscadine Products for Your Health

This book is written for people who know what a muscadine is but may be seeking more knowledge, and for people who have just tasted muscadines and are curious. The book discusses health benefits of the many phytochemicals in muscadines and alerts consumers to new products so that muscadines can become a daily health habit even when fresh fruit is not available.

A Native American Grape- If you live in the Southeastern USA, you may have eaten muscadines all your life. Muscadines are scientifically known as *Vitis rotundifolia* grapes, or more technically, berries. Muscadines are native to SE USA and have naturalized as far north as Delaware. You may have picked them in wood margins or hedgerows as a child. The berries ripen individually within a loose cluster and are not synchronized like bunch grapes. Muscadines were thriving here when the first Europeans arrived. Sir Walter Raleigh remarked upon their prevalence and vigor in 1584-85 [1]. Certainly, the first colonists took advantage of these native grapes and cultivated them. The muscadine is so famous in the state of North Carolina that a "Mother Vine" has become a tourist attraction and cuttings off the "Mother Vine" are sought-after gift items for those who love muscadines.

Native Americans Used the Muscadine for Food and Medicine- Clearly Native Americans enjoyed full benefits of muscadines, muscadine juice and dried (raisined) muscadines. Muscadines were part of the Native American diet in regions wherever they naturalized. The reader can find Cherokee Indian traditional recipes using the online search phrase "possum grapes" or "Cherokee muscadine". "Possum Grapes" are a term used for wild muscadines that grow in traditional Cherokee lands. One such recipe is for Cherokee dumplings. Cherokee and Creek Indians not only ate the whole grapes, but used muscadines in a variety of drinks and poultices [1]. They prepared muscadine juice and added corn meal to make a nutritional beverage. Muscadine dumplings are a favorite among traditional Cherokee recipes [1].

Colonists Prized the Muscadine- These big (5-15 g) grapes were valued highly by the first Europeans who settled on the coasts of what are now the states of Virginia, North Carolina and South Carolina. The scuppernong is a bronze variety of the grape that was found growing wild in North Carolina by hunters around 1755 [2]. Both grow as wild grapes all over the South because birds disperse their seeds and the grapes spring up in most woods, borders and yards. Muscadines naturalized from as far north as Delaware to southern Illinois to northeaster Texas, all through the Gulf of Mexico coastal states back to the SE Atlantic states. Unlike European vinifera grapes, the Vitus rotundifolia varieties are highly adapted to hot humid climates.

Where are muscadines grown commercially? Through the years, horticulturists at major universities and USDA research stations have developed muscadine varieties whose color ranges from bronze to red, purple and black. These cultivars ("cultivated varieties") have been selected for specific characteristics and increased hardiness necessary for commercial success. While muscadines have been domestically cultivated since Colonial times, today's commercial vineyards started in the 1970s and more vineyards are being planted yearly because of the success of this fruit in traditional cotton/tobacco lands that were hard hit by the boll weevil and anti-tobacco legislation. The largest concentrations of muscadine growers are in North Carolina, South Carolina, Georgia, North Florida, Alabama, Mississippi, East Texas and Arkansas. These grapes like the long hot and humid summers of this region of the USA. There are scores of muscadine cultivars. A short list of some of the bronze and purple varieties appears in Table 1.1.

Muscadines are more American than apple pie because they were growing before Johnny Appleseed came around. Here is a recipe that serves as tribute to that history.

All American Muscadine Pie

About 4 cups of muscadines
1 & 1/2 cups of sugar
1 teaspoon of lemon or lime juice
3 tablespoons plain flour
2 tablespoons butter
Your favorite covered pie crust

To prepare, separate hulls from pulp.
Heat pulp to a boil and simmer for 5 minutes.
Press pulp through strainer to separate pulp from seeds.
Discard seeds and mix hulls with pulp.
Mix flour with sugar and lemon/lime juice and blend with hulls
and pulp. Pour muscadine mixture in bottom crust, dot with butter,
cover with top crust. Bake in pre-heated 425°F oven for about 40
minutes.

Serve with vanilla ice cream, a dash of cream sherry or sweet
muscadine wine and some whipped cream and chocolate shavings.

Table 1.1. A Few Commercial Bronze and Purple Muscadine Varieties

Bronze	Purple
Carlos	Black Beauty
Doreen	Cowart
Fry and Early Fry	Ison
Sterling	Jumbo
Summit	Nesbit
Tara	Noble
Triumph	Supreme

Muscadine Products- We write from the viewpoint of researchers who appreciate the muscadine as a powerhouse of natural phytochemicals. We also want you to enjoy this delicious Southern treat as a fresh fruit and in its many product forms that are now available to worldwide markets all year. The muscadine industry has grown considerably in a short 35 years. There is a healthy muscadine wine and juice industry. The nutraceutical and food supplement industries are producing products that allow a hefty daily dose of muscadine phytochemicals in concentrated and convenient forms. In addition, traditional food and beverage products are on the market in record numbers.

Muscadine Product Categories

> **Muscadine whole fruit in season (either purple or bronze)**
> **Muscadine food products (jams, jellies and more)**
> **Muscadine wines (reds or whites, sweet or dry)**
> **Muscadine beverage products (specialty juices)**
> **Muscadine functional food products**
> **Muscadine functional beverage products**
> **Muscadine food supplement products**
> **Muscadine nutraceutical products**

Muscadine Whole Berries- The berries are big, beautiful and luscious. They range in color from yellow green/bronze to purple/black. If you have never eaten a muscadine, they are a grape with incomparable flavors. Muscadines are not a bunch grape, so they are harvested individually when they ripen and are sold fresh at supermarkets, growers' stands and the local farmers'markets in late summer to early fall. There are many cultivars of muscadines being grown commercially right now. They are sometimes referred to as whites or reds. Sometimes these are divided into bronze or purple varieties. In reality, there are muscadines that range from a very light bronze through red range through purple and almost to black. While there are scores of cultivars, popularity with growers is determined by hardiness, fruit quality and the intended use of the fruit after harvest, e.g., fresh fruit market or juice market or winemaking. Bronze varieties are sometimes locally referred to as scuppernongs.

The Great Taste of Muscadines- Muscadines were named for their aromatic flavors. The word is derived from the same root as the French muscatel. Higher alcohols, esters of fatty acids and unique furanones give special aromas and flavors. Various wines taste differently because the relative concentrations at which they occurred in both wines were however different. The more intense peaks appeared in the Noble wine in most cases [3, 4]. We warn you, once you have tasted muscadines, other grapes will never quite compare. Many other grapes will seem like anemic cousins. There is a time-honored method of eating muscadines that every child learns. Bite through the thick skin to get at the rest of the berry, eat the pulp and juice and spit out the seeds. As much as we honor tradition, this practice has to be revisited. To get the full value of the muscadine, skins and seeds need to be chewed well and swallowed. Admittedly these are an acquired taste, therefore many people still grow up and just eat the pulp. New food supplements and nutraceutical products might be the way to get the benefit from the phytochemicals in the seeds. Once you know the medicinal power of those skins and seeds, you'll never throw them out again.

Getting the Full Benefit of Muscadines all Year Round- Fortunately, processed muscadine products give the consumer the medicinal benefit of the muscadine, long after the fruits have disappeared from the fruit stands and produce departments. Muscadine jellies, jams, preserves, pies, assorted sauces (even hot sauces and BBQ sauces), purees and ciders are on the market. Do a website search online using the terms "muscadine products" and you will find many venders who will ship them directly to the consumer. In five minutes you can find hundreds of wholesale, retail and mail order suppliers of these products. Many festivals throughout the SE USA feature muscadine products. Some tourist attractions and resort destinations feature muscadine products year around. The famous Callaway Gardens in Georgia is one such example. Muscadine food products are a wonderful souvenir gift to bring home from the South, or are often used to welcome newcomers and visitors to the South.

Muscadines Wines- A website search online using the terms "muscadine wine" will yield hundreds of wineries and shops in 7-8 states that make both red and white muscadine wines. In just the first 100 sites, you'll not only find merchants selling the wines, but recipes for making muscadine wines and various culinary delights. Muscadine wines are available year round. Most wineries now take personal orders and can ship directly to consumers who may not live in muscadine country.

Some muscadine purple varieties are sent directly to the wineries to begin fermentation with the whole pomace present. As sugars turn to alcohol, many flavonoid and other phenolics (see Chapter 3) are naturally extracted during this process. While the purpose is to extract color and taste molecules into the wine to produce a red wine, this adds additional health benefit to an already medicinal wine. Today, muscadine wine is so popular in SE USA that it is the number one seller at many wineries.

Muscadine Juice- Most muscadines grown commercially are juiced. Some of the juice is bottled and sold as 100% muscadine juice and some is blended for other types of beverages. Muscadine juice is delicious and is a healthy alternative to soda and high fructose corn syrup beverages that are not very good for one's health. Muscadine juice is a good non-alcoholic beverage to serve tee-totalers when wine is being served to other guest at dinner. If you see settlings in some muscadine juices, these are probably due to the content of medicinally beneficial ellagic acid compounds and ellagitannins that form partial precipitates with time. Just as you should eat the skins and seeds of fresh muscadines, you should resuspend these precipitates as you pour a glass of 100% muscadine grape juice to get the full medicinal value.[5]

Muscadine Food Supplement and Nutraceutical Products- The modern food supplement and nutraceutical industry highly values the muscadine skins and seeds left over after the juice has been pressed out of the berries. Perhaps 90% of the medicinal value of the muscadine resides in the skin and seed fractions. The whole pomace can be processed or the skins and seeds can be mechanically separated for individual processing. Each fraction has high nutraceutical value. Dry and powdered, these muscadine fractions yield two benefits. First, the shelf life is long relative to fresh fruit. Second, phytochemicals in the products are much more concentrated in the medicinal phytochemicals than in the whole fruit. This is not an argument against eating whole fruits, it is simply a statement that on a weight basis, one can use these powdered products differently than the whole fruit and get the phytochemical power of the whole fruit in a condensed form. These powders retain the fiber content as well as most of the phytochemical and nutrient composition of the muscadine fresh fraction. And, they are available all year round.

Muscadine Seeds- The seeds can be dried and powdered to produce encapsulated products. Search online using "muscadine grape seed capsules" and you will find retail and mail order sources for these products. Pulverizeing the seed makes it much more digestible because the surface area is increased markedly over whole seed surface area. Remember when we suggested you chew the seeds and skins as you eat the whole fruit? This is to increase the surface area available for the gastrointestinal system to absorb phytochemicals in the seeds or skins. It is not possible or practical to chew skins and seeds long enough to equal what can be done with the milling process in industry. These powders are ideal for increasing the digestibility of the seeds, while leaving the full fiber, oil, and phenolic content in the product.

Muscadine seed extracts are are made to extract a highly concentrated fraction from the seeds that can then be standardized for nutraceutical product or product ingredient use. These extracts are manufactured to contain and concentrate that biomedically most active fraction while decreasing the bulk of the grape seed. Obviously, these extracts do not contain the high fiber content of the pulverized seeds, but will contain the high phenolic and high antioxidant value of the muscadine seed.

Muscadine Skins- Muscadine skins are also highly prized for their medicinal value. Like the seeds, they can be dried and pulverized to produce a finely milled product that retains the high pectin (soluble fiber) of the skins along with the high phenolic content. Pulverized muscadine grape skin products are used as food supplements and are ideal for making smoothies or enhancing the health benefits of various juices. Search online with the phrase " muscadine grape skin" or "muscadine nutraceutical products". **Muscadine skin extracts** are also made by the nutraceutical industry for highly concentrated products. These extracts can be standardized for phenolic content or antioxidant value or any other marker required for nutraceutical product formulation. Again, the basic ingredient is the naturally balanced chemistry of the muscadine. Similarly, **muscadine whole pomace extracts** can be used for food supplement and nutraceutical products.

Muscadine Cosmeceutical Products- Because of their high concentrations of antioxidant phenolic compounds, extracts of muscadines are useful for incorporation into cosmeceutical products. The phenolic fraction has other properties including, anti-bacterial, anti-fungal, anti-UV radiation and anti-cancer that make extracts of muscadines suitable for topical preparations. Search the Internet under "muscadine cosmetic" or "muscadine cosmeceutical" to find manufacturers and distributors of an expanding list of products. These products incorporate a highly concentrated extract of a muscadine fraction into usual cosmetic bases for hand and body lotions, creams, foaming face polish, shampoos etc.

Muscadine Festivals, Tours, Cruises and Entertainment- Search the Internet under "muscadine festivals" and you will find so many festivals showcasing the muscadine in the SE USA for early Fall entertainment. Also, search under "muscadine tours", "muscadine cruises", "muscadine restaurants" and "muscadine theater" for added adventures. Most wineries have tasting sessions that allow the visitor to taste different varieties of wine and other muscadine products.

Muscadine Recipes- Search online "muscadine recipe" or contact a grower or muscadine winery and you'll soon have hundreds of recipes for the whole fruit, fruit puree, fruit juice or wine. Muscadines have been featured on a Cable Food Channel and often appear in seasonal menus of popular household magazines.

The reader can find Cherokee Indian traditional recipes using "possum" grapes, which is another name for wild muscadines. One such recipe is for Cherokee dumplings, in which a dumpling mixture was boiled in muscadine grape juice [1] We tried our own version using powdered muscadine skins in a dumpling mix moistened with bottled muscadine juice from a Georgia vineyard. Delicious!

Cherokee Grape Dumplings

- 1 cup flour
- 1 ½ tsp baking powder
- 2 tsp sugar
- ¼ tsp salt
- 1 tbsp shortening
- ½ cup grape juice

Mix flour, baking powder, sugar, salt and shortening. Add juice and mix into stiff dough. Roll dough very thin on floured board and cut into strips ½" wide (or roll dough in hands and break off pea-sized bits). Drop into boiling grape juice and cook for 10 - 12 minutes.

The website says, "Some Cherokee cooks continue to make their grape dumplings by gathering and cooking wild grapes, or 'possum grapes' instead of grape juice. The John Howard Payne Papers were interviews of elders from 1835. Their knowledge of the old ways tells us that around 1800, a grape dessert was made from boiling the grapes and mashing them and then adding corn meal to make a thick consistency. This seems to be the origin this recipe for grape dumplings that has been enjoyed for the last one hundred years or more."

We have also used muscadine skin powder in biscuits, muffins, pancakes, and cornbread. The skin powder is a wonderful nutraceutical addition to these baked products. In addition, muscadine jams or sauces can be used as a condiment. What a wonderful way to enhance the nutraceutical value of ordinary breakfast foods or juices.

Biomedical Interest in *Vitis* Phytochemicals- In order for a reader to understand the burgeoning biomedical science supporting nutraceutical benefiets of grapes in general, we have prepared a graph of the number of published scientific papers in a PubMed search on Google for grape seed, grape seed extract and grape skins. Figure 1.1 shows that there were a few references each year until 1998, but by 2004, there were hundreds of scientific papers in the literature. There is no sign that the research is slowing down. Muscadines have unique phytochemical profiles and are valued for their seeds, skins, pulp and juice/wine. We call it the "Smarter Grape" because it has an extra set of chromosomes with genes that allow it to create a phytochemical profile with a broader range of nutraceutical potential. Most research that is being done with red grapes and grape seed extracts applies to muscadines as well. However, much more research needs to be done for the All-American Grape.

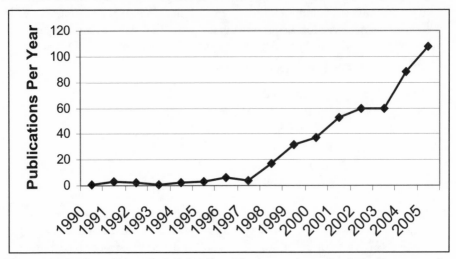

Figure 1.1. Number of biomedical (PubMed) publications per year that deal with grape seed extract and grape skins.

What is a nutraceutical?   The word "nutraceutical" is now becoming a household word. The word was coined by Dr. Stephen DeFelice in a talk at a scientific conference in Italy. Here is his original statement in 1986 [6]:

> "NutraCeutical is the name I have given to a nutritional product - a single entity or combination which includes special diets - that reasonable clinical evidence has shown to have a medical benefit that its manufacturer cannot claim to the public or the physician under present regulatory policy. Making a medical claim for a nutritional product makes that product a drug, according to the prevailing reasoning of the regulatory agency; claims made for drugs must be approved by the government."

Nutraceuticals represent a broad range of products that have medicinal value- The nutraceutical industry manufactures food supplements, functional foods and beverages, herbals, vitamins, nutrients and combination products using natural ingredients. Nutraceuticals are now sold in just about every pharmacy, supermarket, health food store, department store, nutritional supplement store and herbal shop. There are countless online companies that either manufacture bulk ingredients or sell products lines. There are large catalog companies that constitute large distributorships. In addition to FDA regulation of pharmaceuticals, most foods, food additives, beverages, juices and supplements are regulated through the FDA as stipulated by federal code.

FDA Oversight of Dietary Supplements- The food supplement and nutraceutical products manufactured from muscadines will probably all be defined and regulated as dietary supplements by the FDA. It is therefore important to understand how these terms are defined legally. For this, we quote from the FDA's public information on frequently ask questions about food supplements.

"What is a dietary supplement?-Congress defined the term "dietary supplement" in the Dietary Supplement Health and Education Act (DSHEA) of 1994. A dietary supplement is a product taken by mouth that contains a "dietary ingredient" intended to supplement the diet. The "dietary ingredients" in these products may include: vitamins, minerals, herbs or other botanicals, amino acids, and substances such as enzymes, organ tissues, glandulars, and metabolites. Dietary supplements can also be extracts or concentrates, and may be found in many forms such as tablets, capsules, softgels, gelcaps, liquids, or powders. They can also be in other forms, such as a bar, but if they are, information on their label must not represent the product as a conventional food or a sole item of a meal or diet. Whatever their form may be, DSHEA places dietary supplements in a special category under the general umbrella of "foods," not drugs, and requires that every supplement be labeled a dietary supplement."

"What is a "new dietary ingredient" in a dietary supplement?- The Dietary Supplement Health and Education Act (DSHEA) of 1994 defined both of the terms "dietary ingredient" and "new dietary ingredient" as components of dietary supplements. In order for an ingredient of a dietary supplement to be a "dietary ingredient," it must be one or any combination of the following substances:

- a vitamin,
- a mineral,
- an herb or other botanical,
- an amino acid,
- a dietary substance for use by man to supplement the diet by increasing the total dietary intake (e.g., enzymes or tissues from organs or glands), or
- a concentrate, metabolite, constituent or extract.

A "new dietary ingredient" is one that meets the above definition for a "dietary ingredient" and was not sold in the U.S. in a dietary supplement before October 15, 1994."

"What is FDA's role in regulating dietary supplements versus the manufacturer's responsibility for marketing them?"- "In October 1994, the Dietary Supplement Health and Education Act (DSHEA) was signed into law by President Clinton. Before this time, dietary supplements were subject to the same regulatory requirements as were other foods. This new law, which amended the Federal Food, Drug, and Cosmetic Act, created a new regulatory framework for the safety and labeling of dietary supplements.

Under DSHEA, a firm is responsible for determining that the dietary supplements it manufactures or distributes are safe and that any representations or claims made about them are substantiated by adequate evidence to show that they are not false or misleading. This means that dietary supplements do not need approval from FDA before they are marketed. Except in the case of a new dietary ingredient, where pre-market review for safety data and other information is required by law, a firm does not have to provide FDA with the evidence it relies on to substantiate safety or effectiveness before or after it markets its products.

Also, manufacturers do not need to register themselves nor their dietary supplement products with FDA before producing or selling them. Currently, there are no FDA regulations that are specific to dietary supplements that establish a minimum standard of practice for manufacturing dietary supplements. However, FDA intends to issue regulations on good manufacturing practices that will focus on practices that ensure the identity, purity, quality, strength and composition of dietary supplements. At present, the manufacturer is responsible for establishing its own manufacturing practice guidelines to ensure that the dietary supplements it produces are safe and contain the ingredients listed on the label."

"When must a manufacturer or distributor notify FDA about a dietary supplement it intends to market in the U.S.?- The Dietary Supplement Health and Education Act (DSHEA) requires that a manufacturer or distributor notify FDA if it intends to market a dietary supplement in the U.S. that contains a "new dietary ingredient." The manufacturer (and distributor) must demonstrate to FDA why the ingredient is reasonably expected to be safe for use in a dietary supplement, unless it has been recognized as a food substance and is present in the food supply.

There is no authoritative list of dietary ingredients that were marketed before October 15, 1994. Therefore, manufacturers and distributors are responsible for determining if a dietary ingredient is "new", and if it is not, for documenting that the dietary supplements its sells, containing the dietary ingredient, were marketed before October 15, 1994.

"What information must the manufacturer disclose on the label of a dietary supplement?- FDA regulations require that certain information appear on dietary supplement labels. Information that must be on a dietary supplement label includes: a descriptive name of the product stating that it is a "supplement;" the name and place of business of the manufacturer, packer, or distributor; a complete list of ingredients; and the net contents of the product. In addition, each dietary supplement (except for some small volume products or those produced by eligible small businesses) must have nutrition labeling in the form of a "Supplement Facts" panel. This label must identify each dietary ingredient contained in the product."

"Must all ingredients be declared on the label of a dietary supplement?- Yes, ingredients not listed on the "Supplement Facts" panel must be listed in the "other ingredient" statement beneath the panel. The types of ingredients listed there could include the source of dietary ingredients, if not identified in the "Supplement Facts" panel (e.g., rose hips as the source of vitamin C), other food ingredients (e.g., water and sugar), and technical additives or processing aids (e.g., gelatin, starch, colors, stabilizers, preservatives, and flavors). "

"Are dietary supplement serving sizes standardized or are there restrictions on the amount of a nutrient that can be in one serving?- Other than the manufacturer's responsibility to ensure safety, there are no rules that limit a serving size or the amount of a nutrient in any form of dietary supplements. This decision is made by the manufacturer and does not require FDA review or approval."

"Who has the responsibility for ensuring that a dietary supplement is safe?- By law (DSHEA), the manufacturer is responsible for ensuring that its dietary supplement products are safe before they are marketed. Unlike drug products that must be proven safe and effective for their intended use before marketing, there are no provisions in the law for FDA to "approve" dietary supplements for safety or effectiveness before they reach the consumer. Also unlike drug products, manufacturers and distributors of dietary supplements are not currently required by law to record, investigate or forward to FDA any reports they receive of injuries or illnesses that may be related to the use of their products. Under DSHEA, once the product is marketed, FDA has the responsibility for showing that a dietary supplement is "unsafe," before it can take action to restrict the product's use or removal from the marketplace."

"Do manufacturers or distributors of dietary supplements have to tell FDA or consumers what evidence they have about their product's safety or what evidence they have to back up the claims they are making for them?- No, except for rules described above that govern "new dietary ingredients," there is no provision under any law or regulation that FDA enforces that requires a firm to disclose to FDA or consumers the information they have about the safety or purported benefits of their dietary supplement products. Likewise, there is no prohibition against them making this information available either to FDA or to their customers. It is up to each firm to set its own policy on disclosure of such information.

"How can consumers inform themselves about safety and other issues related to dietary supplements?- It is important to be well informed about products before purchase. Because it is often difficult to know what information is reliable and what is questionable, consumers may first want to contact the manufacturer about the product they intend to purchase. In addition, to help consumers in their search to be better informed, FDA is providing the following sites: *Tips For The Savvy Supplement User:* Making

Informed Decisions And Evaluating Information located here: http://www.cfsan.fda.gov/~dms/ds-savvy.html (includes information on how to evaluate research findings and health information on-line) and Claims That Can Be Made for Conventional Foods and Dietary Supplements -- http://www.cfsan.fda.gov/~dms/hclaims.html, (provides information on what types of claims can be made for dietary supplements)."

"What is FDA's oversight responsibility for dietary supplements?-
Because dietary supplements are under the "umbrella" of foods, FDA's Center for Food Safety and Applied Nutrition (CFSAN) is responsible for the agency's oversight of these products. FDA's efforts to monitor the marketplace for potential *illegal* products (that is, products that may be unsafe or make false or misleading claims) include obtaining information from inspections of dietary supplement manufacturers and distributors, the Internet, consumer and trade complaints, occasional laboratory analyses of selected products, and adverse events associated with the use of supplements that are reported to the agency."

"Does FDA routinely analyze the content of dietary supplements?-
In that FDA has limited resources to analyze the composition of food products, including dietary supplements, it focuses these resources first on public health emergencies and products that may have caused injury or illness. Enforcement priorities then go to products thought to be unsafe or fraudulent or in violation of the law. The remaining funds are used for routine monitoring of products pulled from store shelves or collected during inspections of manufacturing firms. The agency does not analyze dietary supplements before they are sold to consumers. The manufacturer is responsible for ensuring that the "Supplement Facts" label and ingredient list are accurate, that the dietary ingredients are safe, and that the content matches the amount declared on the label. FDA does not have resources to analyze dietary supplements sent to the agency by consumers who want to know their content. Instead, consumers may contact the manufacturer or a commercial laboratory for an analysis of the content."

"Is it legal to market a dietary supplement product as a treatment or cure for a specific disease or condition?- No, a product sold as a dietary supplement and promoted on its label or in labeling* as a treatment, prevention or cure for a specific disease or condition would be considered an unapproved-- and thus illegal--drug. To maintain the product's status as a dietary supplement, the label and labeling must be consistent with the provisions in the Dietary Supplement Health and Education Act (DSHEA) of 1994.

*Labeling refers to the label as well as accompanying material that is used by a manufacturer to promote and market a specific product."

"Who validates claims and what kinds of claims can be made on dietary supplement labels?- FDA receives many consumer inquiries about the validity of claims for dietary supplements, including product labels, advertisements, media, and printed materials. The responsibility for ensuring the validity of these claims rests with the manufacturer, FDA, and, in the case of advertising, with the Federal Trade Commission.

By law, manufacturers may make three types of claims for their dietary supplement products: health claims, structure/function claims, and nutrient content claims. Some of these claims describe: the link between a food substance and disease or a health-related condition; the intended benefits of using the product; or the amount of a nutrient or dietary substance in a product. Different requirements generally apply to each type of claim, and are described in more detail here: (http://www.cfsan.fda.gov/~dms/hclaims.html)."

"Why do some supplements have wording (a disclaimer) that says: "This statement has not been evaluated by the FDA. This product is not intended to diagnose, treat, cure, or prevent any disease"?

This statement or "disclaimer" is required by law (DSHEA) when a manufacturer makes a structure/function claim on a dietary supplement label. In general, these claims describe the role of a nutrient or dietary ingredient intended to affect the structure or function of the body. The manufacturer is responsible for ensuring the accuracy and truthfulness of these claims; they are not approved by FDA. For this reason, the law says that if a dietary supplement label includes such a claim, it must state in a "disclaimer" that FDA has not evaluated this claim. The disclaimer must also state that this product is not intended to "diagnose, treat, cure or prevent any disease," because only a drug can legally make such a claim."

"How are advertisements for dietary supplements regulated?

The Federal Trade Commission (FTC) regulates advertising, including infomercials, for dietary supplements and most other products sold to consumers. FDA works closely with FTC in this area, but FTC's work is directed by different laws. Advertising and promotional material received in the mail are also regulated under different laws and are subject to regulation by the U.S. Postal Inspection Service."

The FTC states: "Marketers of dietary supplements should be familiar with the requirements under both DSHEA and the FTC Act that labeling and advertising claims be truthful, not misleading and substantiated. The FTC approach generally requires that claims be backed by sound, scientific evidence, but also provides flexibility in the precise amount and type of support necessary. This flexibility allows advertisers to provide truthful information to consumers about the benefits of supplement products, and at the same time, preserves consumer confidence by curbing unsubstantiated, false, and misleading claims. To ensure compliance with FTC law, supplement advertisers should follow two important steps: 1) careful drafting of advertising claims with particular attention to how claims are qualified and what express and implied messages are actually conveyed to consumers; and 2) careful review of the support for a claim to make sure it is scientifically sound, adequate in the context of the surrounding body of evidence, and relevant to the specific product and claim advertised."

Role for Muscadines, Muscadine Food Supplements and Nutraceutical Products for Health Maintenance and Disease Prevention- In the following chapters, the authors have digested a very large body of biomedical literature concerning the phytochemicals in muscadines. We particularly emphasize the phenolic compounds for their health value because these compounds are not well known by the public. We introduce specific phytochemicals and summarize relevant biomedical literature concerning their nutraceutical value. In some instances, we let the reader know how large are the databases and show the reader how to search the primary biomedical literature using Entrez Pubmed from the National Library of Medicine. This allows the reader to better evaluate the validity of statements in mass media or online sources.

Our goal as scientists is to discuss biomedical reasons for following the recommendations of nearly every major public health agency, health advocacy group or authorities from nutrition science, functional genomics, pharmacognosy, pharmacology, preventive medicine, complementary medicine, integrative medicine, alternative medicine, natural medicine and nutritional and dietetic counselers. We emphasize the importance of a diet high in phytochemicals for the prevention, amelioration, treatment (integrated with modern medicine) cure or reversal (integrated with modern medicine) that influence the health of many body systems. This is true whether the body is healthy and trying to stay healthy; whether the body is getting unhealthy and is trying to regain health; or, whether the body is unhealthy and needs to ameliorate or reverse the disease state. We have specifically directed our chapters to those chronic disease states that plague our society and which are known to be prevented or influenced by a diet high in phytochemical choices. Such diets can be composed from a range of highly colored plant parts, fruits, berries, vegetables, barks, roots, leaves, stems, seeds, nuts, legumes, pulses and grains.

We urge the reader to read the suggestions and cautionary notes from the FDA. However, FDA does no research, so also read the recommendations of public health authorities and individuals who assert that diet and lifestyle choices do help people 'prevent, ameliorate, treat, cure or reverse' some of the chronic diseases that plague our society. These authoritative sources encourage us to prevent heart disease and atherosclerosis, prediabetes, diabetes, metabolic syndrome, cancers, inflammatory diseases, gastrointestinal diseases and neurological diseases.

It should be obvious to the reader why food supplement and nutraceutical manufacturers are not allowed to say very much about their products. The FDA (see pg 13) states that any " product sold as a dietary supplement and promoted on its label or in labeling* as a treatment, prevention or cure for a specific disease or condition would be considered an unapproved--and thus illegal--drug." It is also true that the FDA and FTC will not allow any fruit or vegetable to be marketed for its value in preventing, treating, ameliorating or reversing (curing) any specific disease or condition unless FDA has specifically approved a health claim. Unlike the NIH and CDC, the FDA and FTC are not research agencies, rather, they are regulatory agencies. Clearly, with industry operating within these regulatory constraints, consumers need to be self-educated.

This book is written to emphasize muscadines as phytochemically powerful choices within a maximally healthy diet. We believe in disease prevention, treatment, amelioration and reversal. We hope that what we say about muscadines will prompt the reader to make informed choices that will consistently improve the nutraceutical quality of the total diet. Dietary and lifestyle choices are paramount to achieving maximal health and longevity.

Web Resources

The Cherokee Nation culture and food traditions, http://www.cherokee.org/Culture/CulturePage.asp?ID=48

Food and Drug Administration (FDA) Dietary Supplement Information, http://www.cfsan.fda.gov/~dms/supplmnt.html

FDA Dietary Ingredient information, http://www.cfsan.fda.gov/~dms/ds-ingrd.html.

FDA Supplement Labeling, http://www.cfsan.fda.gov/~lrd/fr97923a.html.

FDA Health Claims, http://www.cfsan.fda.gov/~dms/hclaims.html

Federal Trade Commission (FTC) http://www.ftc.gov/bcp/menu-health.htm.

FTC Advertising Guidelines: http://www.ftc.gov/bcp/conline/pubs/buspubs/dietsupp.htm

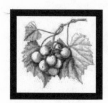

Chapter 2-

Muscadines – The Smarter Grape!

Muscadines are hardy grapes that thrive under conditions that kill European grapes. They are classified as a separate species of grape that does not readily hybridize with the European stock [7]. Geneticists have learned that muscadines have an extra pair of chromosomes. Whereas European grapes and the American Concord grape have 19 pairs of chromosomes, the muscadine has 20 pairs of chromosomes [8]. The extra pair of chromosomes means muscadines have more genetic information. This surely accounts for the ability to thrive in the high heat and humidity of SE USA.

Chromosomes contain genes that are the genetic blueprint for enzymes and other proteins. The additional genes almost certainly allow muscadines to produce its unique balance of phytochemicals, e.g., the ellagic acid family of compounds that are in muscadines that are virtually absent in other grapes. Muscadine genes encode all the different processes that allow this grape to develop a thicker skin to protect it against heat, UV radiation, humidity, insects and fungi. The extra genetic information qualifies the muscadine as the "smarter grape". The specific genes on this extra pair of chromosomes have not been identified. While the "adaptogenic" phytochemicals are there to help the muscadine, these compounds happen to be medicinal once people ingest muscadines.

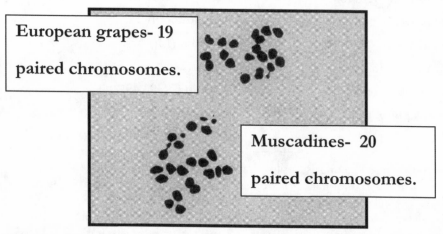

Figure 2.1. A set of chromosomes from European grapes (top) shows 19 chromosomes (large dark spots) from each seed parent. Muscadines have 20 chromosomes (bottom left). Redrawn from [8] with permission.

What makes a muscadine medicinal? Let's take an inventory of the phytochemicals in muscadines that contribute to their nutraceutical or medicinal value. While the muscadine contains a range of vitamins, oils, fiber, sugars and proteins that are nutritious, the greater value of the muscadine to the nutraceutical industry is in the phenolic fraction. Several analytical studies on muscadines reveal a profile of potent phytochemicals. The phenolic fraction alone will contain the following phytochemicals, all of which have medicinal value. While the muscadine literature is growing, it is still very small. In comparison, the number of biomedical papers that have been written on the phytochemicals in muscadines is enormous and very supportive of the nutraceutical power of this smarter grape. Below is a list of many of the phytochemicals in muscadines and we searched the biomedical databases for the number of citations for each. This search was done as the first muscadines came into harvest season in August 2005. The sheer volume of published research attests to the scientific interest in these compounds. The reader can go to Google, type in Pubmed and do an Entrez Pubmed search using the following search terms. If you find even more citations than below, you can judge how fast this field is growing

Table 2.1. Muscadine Phytochemicals. PubMed Biomedical Literature Search (Phytochemical and number of research citations)

•Ellagic Acid (601)	• Quercetin (4306)
•Resveratrol (1081)	•Tartaric Acid (754)
•Chlorogenic Acid (783)	•Cyanidin (322)
•Caffeic Acid (1292)	•Peonidin (85)
•Cinnamic Acid (589)	•Delphinidin (150)
•Epicatechin (2844)	•Petunidin (49)
•Gallic Acid (3091)	•Malvidin (121)
•Geraniol (383)	•Pectin (2440)
•Coumaric Acid (386)	•Vitamin C (30,249)
•Kaempferol (1027)	•Anthocyanidins (1467)
•Myricetin (372)	•OPCs Oligomeric Procyanidins (93)

Among these chemicals, only vitamin C and pectin (a dietary fiber) are recognized as traditional nutrients, and only vitamin C is essential. While the above list will surely expand as more analytical chemists study the muscadine, it already represents a staggering number of biomedically active phytochemicals with well-known beneficial effects. Together, the list itself makes a good argument for eating muscadines, muscadine products and potent extracts of muscadines in nutraceutical products. Incidentally, Dr. Betty Ector stated that muscadines have more dietary fiber than oats [9]. The fiber acts as a delivery system that takes the phytochemicals to the gastrointestinal tract where they are needed. Powdered muscadine skin and seed products also are extremely high in dietary fiber content while they deliver the phytochemical power of the muscadine.

Muscadines Fit Into New US Dietary Guidelines- While regulatory agencies are still in a worldwide quandary over how to handle nutraceuticals, most of us realize that many of these products are food supplements to replete a modern diet that has become more stocked with available calories, but is depleted in phytochemicals necessary to maintain optimal health. In 2005 there was yet another revision of the official US dietary guidelines. New U.S. dietary guidelines and a new Food Guide Pyramid (actually a series of pyramids) were announced. These get revised regularly, so sometimes these announcements don't have much fanfare. This time, the appointed committee of experts got it almost right. The new pyramid is a rainbow of colors that spans whole grains, vegetables, fruits, dairy products, meat and beans. Whole grapes are prominently displayed, and the pyramid rainbow ends in phytochemical purple. We'd like to think of this as muscadine purple. Notice that the recommendations are largely for whole foods. The color-coding is designed to let the consumer make the very best choices from a range of fruits and vegetables that will add the very best phytochemical profile to the diet.

Basic Nutrient Profile of Muscadines- Muscadines are low in fat with moderate levels of protein and carbohydrate. The carbohydrates include fructose, glucose and sucrose-remember that fructose does not raise blood glucose. There is very little sodium and a healthy amount of potassium. A

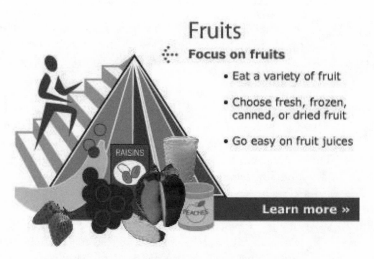

Figure 2.2. A portion of the 2005 U.S.D.A. Food Guide Pyramid that includes fruits, grapes, and other berries. Source: USDA Food Guide Pyramid: http://www.mypyramid.gov.

Table 2.2. Essential Nutrients in Muscadine Grapes per 100 g Serving.
Data compiled by Dr. Betty Ector [9].

Nutrient	Bronze-skinned	Dark-skinned
Protein	0.5 g	0.5 g
Fat	0.4 g	0.4 g
Carbohydrate	12 g	14 g
Energy	68 Calories	76 Calories
Sodium	5 mg	7 mg
Calcium	17 mg	24 mg
Potassium	163 mg	167 mg
Magnesium	5 mg	5 mg
Vitamin C	7 mg	6 mg
Dietary Fiber	3 g	3 g
Soluble Fiber	1 g	1 g

serving of this size contains 10% of the recommended amount of vitamin C and is a good source of fiber [9], which helps lower cholesterol. To put this in perspective, 100 g of cooked oats contains less than 2 g of dietary fiber!

Muscadines are technically a berry fruit that can provide the phytochemicals deemed beneficial in the purple to red range. The new Food Guide Pyramid shows raisins (dried grapes) as an example of a dried whole food product that is a rich source of antioxidants. The pyramid advises a person to "go easy" on fruit juices. This is well meant, but just a little off base. Many people drink "fruit drinks", not totally natural fruit juices. The fruit drinks are usually formulated with a certain percentage of natural fruit juice or concentrate, but this includes high fructose corn syrup sweeteners and food additives for palatability, flavor, color and shelf life. If that is what you are drinking, "go easy" indeed. In fact, eliminating that type of fruit beverage would be a good health decision. On the other hand, if you are drinking natural fruit juices, like 100% muscadine juice, you are getting a phytochemical feast and this is an excellent replacement for artificial juices or soft drink products. Try putting

100% muscadine juice on your list of other healthy choices like 100% orange juice, vegetable juices and tomato juice. One can enjoy a range of deeply colored juices that provide the phytochemicals in the color-coded diet selections of the new food guidelines. If these juices are balanced out with high fiber foods, juice drinkers will compensate for the loss of the fruit fiber.

How Much Is A Serving Of Muscadines? With the new 2005 Dietary Guidelines, the recommendation for grapes is based on 5 to 9 servings of fruit and vegetables a day. The Centers for Disease Control recommends 1-½ cups as a serving for a 2,000 Calorie diet. This amount typically contains about 90 calories, 23 g of natural fruit sugars, 270 mg of potassium, no sodium, and 25% of daily vitamin C plus abundant phytochemicals. Grape sugars are a mixture of glucose and fructose, with a small amount of sucrose [10]. Fructose is the same sugar that is found in honey, and it gives muscadine juice its sweet flavor. For muscadine juice, a serving size is considered to be 1 cup (8 oz).

Color Codes to Choose Nutraceutical Power Foods- When composing a daily diet of 5-9 servings of fruits and vegetables, it is left to the consumer to choose from what is available. It is possible for the consumer to make power choices from various available choices that will maximize the health benefits fully. Let's take fruit choices. The consumer can do this easily by first choosing very deeply colored fruits to maximize the phytochemical content range. A table is shown on the next page to give you an idea of the chemicals associated with each of these colors of fruits and vegetables.

There are many kinds of phytochemicals in every plant, and often the chemicals are concentrated in the peels or rinds, as is the case for the bioflavonoids in citrus. The table gives examples of why it is important to select foods from across the color rainbow at every meal. Consider the color purple in grapes. All grapes are good for your health, but muscadines grapes are very powerful choices because of the high phytochemical content their skins and seeds. Relative to many other grapes, they have an unique range of chemicals.

Many of the health benefits of deeply colored fruits and vegetables are in the compounds that give color and taste to the plant. Some plants are just richer sources than others, as shown in Table 2.3.

Table 2.3. The color spectrum of foods with examples of phytochemicals that are often associated with foods of that color.

Color	Foods
Red (Lycopene, beta carotene, other carotenoids)	Tomatoes, pasta sauce, tomato-based soups and juices, pink grapefruit and watermelon
Red to Purple (Anthocyanins, resveratrol, flavonoids)	Muscadines and purple grapes, muscadine juices and wines, other red wines and grape juices, raisins, prunes, cranberries, blueberries, blackberries, strawberries, red peppers, plums, cherries, eggplant, red beets
Orange (Carotenoids)	Carrots, mangoes, apricots, cantaloupe, sweet potatoes, acorn squash, winter squash
Orange to Yellow (Flavonoids)	Oranges, orange juice, tangerines, yellow grapefruit, lemons, limes, citrus zest, nectarines, peaches, papaya, pineapple
Yellow to Green (Chlorophyll)	Spinach, collards, mustard or turnip greens, romaine, yellow corn, avocado, green peas and beans, peppers, cucumber, kiwi, honeydew, zucchini
Green (Chlorophyll, sulphoraphane, indole-3-carbinol)	Broccoli, Brussels sprouts, cabbage, cauliflower, Chinese cabbage, kale
Green to White (Quercetin, allicin)	Onions, garlic, leeks, celery, asparagus, artichokes, endive, chives, mushrooms, apples

Look at the photo composite (Fig. 2.3) and you can see that the big purple muscadines are deeply colored but the table grapes are not. What you cannot see is that the muscadines have a very thick skin vs the very thin skin on the table grape. The skin of the muscadine (of both the bronze and purple varieties) is packed with, high antioxidant phytochemicals with high nutraceutical value. Obviously the table grapes have been cultivated for their thin skins and this selection decreases their nutraceutical value. Also, the table grapes are seedless. This may have certain appeal to consumers who don't like to eat seeds or who were taught to spit them out as they eat grapes. Muscadines have high antioxidant, high nutraceutical value seeds. While there may be many reasons to purchase a seedless table grape, nutraceutical value is not one of them. Many of the beneficial phytochemicals are in the grape skins and seeds. It is therefore important to eat those skins and seeds and chew them well for better digestion and absorption. One of the compounds in muscadines that distinguishes them from cousins in the grape family are their range of ellagic acid-containing compounds. Ellagic acid (and its many derivatives including

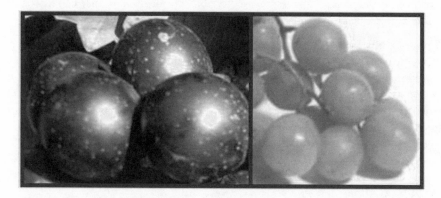

PURPLE MUSCADINES   SEEDLESS TABLE GRAPES

Figure 2.3. Comparison of muscadine grapes with typical table grapes.

ellagitannins) exist in the muscadines, but not to any significant amount in other supermarket grapes. These compounds are not only powerful antioxidants, but have been shown to have potent anti-cancer properties. Similarly, the juices of various grapes contain different ranges of phytochemicals. Ellagic acid compounds from muscadines also appear in muscadine juice fraction [11].

The 2005 U.S. Dietary Guidelines- The new Dietary Guidelines are based on important human epidemiologic and clinical nutritional studies that show diets higher in fresh fruits, vegetables and whole grains will lower blood pressure. One large human clinical prospective study is called the Dietary Approach to Stop Hypertension or DASH diet. The original idea was that an improved balance with less table salt (sodium) and more potassium would reduce blood pressure. It did [12-20]. The DASH diet also increased dietary magnesium. Magnesium is much higher in whole grains than in highly processed grains. This increased magnesium intake contributed to the decrease in blood pressure.

The Dietary Guidelines recommend 4-5 servings per day of fruit/berries for those on a typical 2000-calorie daily meal plan. Most men and active teenagers need more energy than this, so 6 servings would be appropriate. Muscadines would be an excellent choice. One dietary supplement muscadine grape skin product on the market is formulated for smoothies. Muscadines are an excellent source of potassium and are naturally low in sodium. While these ions are not the phytochemicals that we consider the nutraceutical fraction of muscadines, you can understand how these may work well into an anti-cardiovascular disease prevention diet. Muscadines are so large that one "official" serving is just a few grape berries. Round out daily fruit and vegetable selections with other colors (apples, oranges, and bananas) and you are on your way to maintaining healthy blood pressure and reducing high blood pressure.

For those on high blood pressure medication, a good DASH diet can lower the amount of medication needed to maintain a healthy blood pressure.

Whole Foods Haven't Lost Their Phytochemicals- The phytochemicals in a whole food diet are collectively antioxidant and anti-inflammatory. These activities help defend against age-related problems. Emphasizing whole foods also helps maintain a healthy weight because it is bulky and a person feels satisfied sooner. Synthetic foods tend to be composed of the cheapest possible ingredients reconstructed into a form with texture and artificial additives and colorants. Synthetic foods do not have the holistic balance of chemicals that exist in whole foods. Remember that a whole vegetable, a whole fruit, a whole grain or whole seeds, nuts or legumes have all the chemicals supporting life, and in proportions that exist in a living system.

Finally, the US Dietary Guidelines say nothing about the use of nutraceutical products to enhance this suggested diet. Vitamins, minerals, food supplements and nutraceutical products can significantly optimize even these guideline diets. Issues may arise concerning altered nutritional content of modern whole foods because of changes in plant breeding, agricultural practices, food processing and food storage concerns are not addressed in the guidelines. A savvy consumer will take the guidelines as a background and then optimize choices within those guidelines.

National Cancer Institute Guidelines. What about cancer prevention? The National Cancer Institute (NCI) and other agencies that are leading the research effort to prevent and treat cancer have supported the 5-A-Day program for fruits and vegetables for years. In many parts of the United States, people consume fewer than 1-2 servings a day, even counting French fries and iceberg lettuce as vegetables. Why? Because cancer experts know that cumulative research at the epidemiological, clinical research and basic science research indicates a diet higher in a range of fruits and vegetables with whole grains, legumes and unsalted nuts and healthy fats lower the incidence of our most prevalant cancers. Here is what the cancer experts recommend:

"Healthy food choices and physical activity may help reduce the risk of cancer. The following diet and fitness guidelines may help reduce the risk of cancer:"

- Eat a plant-based diet. Eat at least 5 servings of fruit and vegetables daily. Include beans in the diet and eat grain products (such as cereals, breads, and pasta) several times daily.
- Choose foods low in fat.
- Choose foods low in salt.
- Get to and stay at a healthy weight.
- Be at least moderately active for 30 minutes on most days of the week.
- Limit alcoholic drinks.
- Prepare and store food safely.
- Do not use tobacco in any form.

National Cancer Institute (NCI) Recommendations for Preventing Specific Cancers:

Lung Cancer
- Eating more than 5 servings per day of fruits and vegetables may reduce the risk of lung cancer.

Prostate Cancer
- Diets high in saturated fat and meat or animal fat may increase the risk of advanced prostate cancer.
- Taking daily vitamin E supplements may reduce the risk of death from prostate cancer.
- Taking daily beta-carotene supplements may reduce the chance of dying from prostate cancer. Taking beta-carotene supplements is not advised for smokers, however, as it may increase their risk of developing prostate cancer.

Breast Cancer
- High-calorie, high-fat diets may increase the risk of recurrence.
- Drinking beer may increase the risk of recurrence and death.
- Obesity (having too much body fat) may increase the risk of recurrence.
- Lack of physical activity may increase the risk of recurrence.
- Taking vitamin C above the RDA may reduce the risk of recurrence.
- A diet high in vegetables and fruits may reduce the risk of recurrence.
- A diet rich in foods that contain beta-carotene (such as dark orange vegetables and fruits) may reduce the risk of death from breast cancer.

Colon Cancer
- A long-term diet rich in whole grains may reduce the risk of colon cancer.

Esophageal and Gastric Cancer
- A diet rich in cereal fiber may reduce the risk of gastric cancer.
- Taking daily supplements of vitamins C and E and beta-carotene may reduce the risk of esophageal cancer.

Paradox: FDA vs National Cancer Institute- We hope that the reader has noticed a certain paradox. Namely, the U.S. Food and Drug Administration maintains that any substance intended to prevent, treat or ameliorate a disease is a drug. Meantime, the National Cancer Institute and every other health research arm of the National Institutes of Health is saying that what you need to do to prevent cancers is to eat more fruits and vegetables and other whole foods. Just about every agency blames part of the higher rates of cancers on modern diets and inactive life styles. Many cancer experts suggest a highly plant-based whole food diet even if the consumer is not vegetarian. Muscadine grapes and grape products are excellent choices to fit with any healthy eating plan. They should be eaten along with all these other healthful foods. Muscadine nutraceutical products and food supplements provide a daily enhancement to this diet. In conclusion, muscadines and scuppernongs are clearly excellent choices for a healthy diet.

Web Resources

U.S. Dietary Guidelines 2005: http://www.healthierus.gov/dietaryguidelines

USDA Food Guide Pyramid: http://www.mypyramid.gov

National Cancer Institute:
http://www.cancer.gov/cancertopics/pdq/supportivecare/nutrition

http://www.5aday.com/html/phytochem/pic_home.php

Centers for Disease Control:
http://www.cdc.gov/nccdphp/dnpa/5ADay/month/grapes.htm

Five-A-Day Program: http://www.5aday.com/html/phytochem/pic_home.p

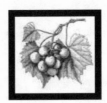

Chapter 3-

Phytochemical Power of Muscadine Grapes, Skins, Seeds and Extracts

The most powerful antioxidants in muscadines are concentrated in the skins and seeds, but the mixture of contributing phytochemicals differs in these two parts. The antioxidants in grape skin act as natural sunscreens, ward off insects, and prevent infection by viruses, bacteria and molds. In nature, the role of the seed is to produce new grape vines, so it also must be protected against being eaten and digested. The seeds are tough and are spread by birds and other animals that eat grapes. Muscadine pulp and juice also have nutraceutical value in addition to high Vitamin C content. There is great interest in the health benefits of grape seed extract and also grape skins [21-37].

Muscadine Antioxidant Power- The typical American consumes only 2-3 servings of fruit and vegetables per day, and this yields about 5,700 units of total antioxidant power [38]. One cup of muscadine grapes (160 grams) contains about 8,000 units of antioxidant power, so a single serving of muscadine grapes would more than double the average person's antioxidant intake. This puts muscadines and scuppernongs in the elite list of powerful antioxidant foods that also includes blueberries, blackberries, cranberries, raspberries and cereal bran. The antioxidants are concentrated in muscadine grape skins and seeds, and 1 gram of these dried nutraceutical products can add about 600-1100 units of antioxidant power.

Vitamin C (ascorbic acid) is the best-known antioxidant, but it is just one of many antioxidant compounds that are found in muscadines and other fruits and berries. It contributes less than 30% to total antioxidant values in most fruits. It may even be added to some commercially fruit juices. Muscadine juice is naturally a good source of vitamin C. Many of the other antioxidant substances in muscadines have considerable range of bioactivities beyond their antioxidant capacity.

Different Tests for Antioxidant Capacity- Three common tests used to evaluate and compare antioxidant values are the **ORAC, FRAP** and **TEAC** assays. ORAC is the Oxygen Radical Absorbance Capcity assay. FRAP is the Ferric Reducing Ability of Plasma assay. TEAC is the Trolox Equivalent Antioxidant Capacity assay. It is important for the consumer to realize that these are simple tests of total antioxidant activity. They are different tests and have different unit values and these cannot be mixed and matched. An excellent paper was written that compared the ORAC, FRAP and TEAC assays on phenolic extracts of fruits and vegetables, as well as Vitamin C. [39] The study showed that using easch assay, there was a direct correlation between ORAC, FRAP and TEAC units and the phenolic fractions tested. The same was true when Vitamin C was tested.

Each of these tests is valid for the phytochemistry of the muscadine. Remember that these tests just indicate the total antioxidant activity of a whole mixture of substances in the test tube. The tests do not tell you which substances are contributing to that value. Those data are derived from more analytical studies taking into account the amount and antioxidant contribution of each individual chemical. Obviously, this is not done regularly. Many laboratories do try to separate out the total phenolic fraction vs the Vitamin C content for example. Other laboratories will further characterize the phenolic fraction. What is important is that these are *in vitro* tests and should not be equated with *in vivo* effects.

ORAC values are usually given as micromoles of Trolox (a vitamin E-like antioxidant) equivalents (per g of fruit or per liter of extract (or mg TE/kg). The higher the number, the greater is the antioxidant power of the fruit or berry. Dr. Ronald Prior's laboratory has now provided ORAC values per serving of common U.S. fruits and vegetables (edible portions).

Don't Get Confused by ORAC, FRAP and TEAC Values- The antioxidant capacity or ORAC varies among different fruits and berries, but it is misleading to compare numbers from different sources. This is because published numbers depend on whether seeds and skins have been removed, how the antioxidants were extracted from dry matter, and the skill of the analytical laboratory. For example, one of the original reports on ORAC in fruits and vegetables provided a value of 7 units per gram for red grapes and 15 units for strawberries [40]. Another report stated that blueberries range from 4.6 to 30 units per gram [41]. However, a later report from the same laboratory showed ORAC values of wine grapes from 37 to 135 units, compared to 52-139 for blueberries and 62-82 for blackberries [42]. These differences may be explained by improvements in methods. The ORAC test has evolved with time and now it is common to see both a lipophilic and a hydrophilic ORAC value given. The reader needs to understand that inconsistency exists in nature from crop to crop, variety to variety, environment condition to environment condistion. It gets more confused when numbers are mixed and matched and compared between labs and across different methodologies. Unfortunately, ORAC is sometimes used as a marketing tool for comparing one fruit to another. A product can have a high ORAC value but no phytochemicals if it just is spiked with Vitamin C. So, the greater interest after one finds that berries have high ORAC value is to look at the specific chemistry contributing to that ORAC value. This is also true of FRAP and TEAC assays.

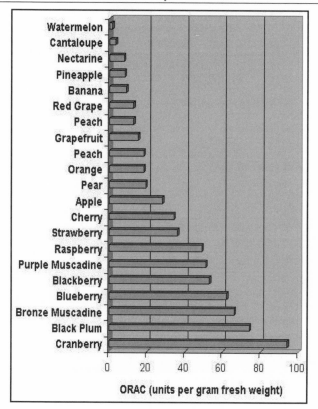

Figure 3.1. ORAC values for a variety of berries and other fruits. Notice that muscadines have ORAC values similar to other power fruits like raspberries and blueberries.

Muscadine ORAC Values- ORAC values are only a beginning but let's look at some typical ORAC values for muscadine fractions or products. How do muscadine grapes compare with other fruits? Typical ORAC values for whole muscadines range from about 33-66 units per gram of fresh fruit. This range of values overlaps the ranges noted for blueberries, blackberries, plums, oranges and grapefruit. Wu et al. (2004) have provided an excellent summary of ORAC values in common fruits, berries and vegetables [38]. Wine and juice and whole fruit may appear lower, but remember that a serving is many times this value.

Antioxidant Values In A Range Of Fruits- Figure 3.1 shows a wide range of ORAC values per gram of fresh fruit. This is not meant to start a fruit war over which fruit packs the highest ORAC. These are fresh or "wet" weights, so dried, raisined, powdered or extracted fruits would be expected to have much higher values per unit weight. Again, the ORAC value is just an antioxidant measure in a test tube. What is important is what the chemicals can do in for human health. All of these fruits are excellent choices for health. The chart really emphasizes that on a weight basis, the berry crops are loaded with antioxidant power.

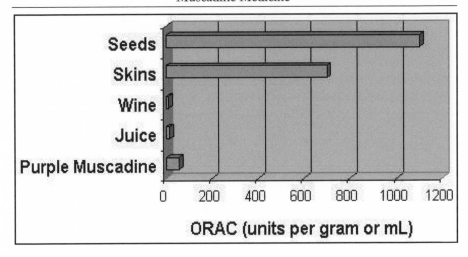

Figure 3.2. Typical ORAC values for muscadine grape parts per gram or mL. Because servings of grapes, juice or wine are at least 100 g or mL, the amount per serving is quite high for all these products.

Antioxidants in Muscadine Juices and Wines- The amount of antioxidant power found in muscadine juices and wines depends on whether a cold or hot extraction procedure was used and on length of storage. Cold processing, which is widely used for commercial operations, yields juices with about 5-14 units per milliliter and wines with about 5-10 units per mL. However, a hot extraction increases these values to about 40-60 units per mL [43]. A cup of cold-processed juice will add 1200 to 2400 units of antioxidant power to a person's diet, and a cup of hot processed juice could add almost 10,000 units, more than double the average intake! Servings for wine are smaller (6 ounces or 180 mL) but would add anywhere from 1,800 to 10,000 units of antioxidant power.

Muscadine berries are about 50% pulp, 40% grape skins, and 10% grape seeds [44]. The phenolic antioxidants and the greatest ORAC capacity are concentrated in the skins and seeds. For this reason, when juice is prepared, most of the ORAC value from the whole grape is found in seeds and skins and less is in the juice. This makes the grape skins and grape seeds highly desirable as nutraceutical sources of antioxidants and polyphenolics. For example, fresh muscadine juice contains about 5-23 TE units per liter compared to 23-66 units per g fresh grapes. The skins have about 422-700 TE units per g, and the seeds have about 667-1100 units per g [44]. Therefore, the amount of total antioxidants in a gram of grape seeds is about twice as much as in grape skins, 10 times as much as in whole grapes, and at least 30 times as much as in the juice.

Muscadine skins have about 6-8 times as much antioxidant capacity as whole blueberries. The muscadine seeds have more than 10 times as much antioxidant capacity as blueberries. The ORAC values for various blueberries ranges from

52-139 TE units per g compared to 62-82 for blackberries. Now, blueberries and blackberries are excellent choices in daily fruit intake. Our point is that dried and powdered muscadine seeds, skins or pomace are powerful sources of nutraceuticals..

Muscadine Wines- The health value of wine has been known for centuries. In modern times, the health benefits of wines have been documented with many excellent studies. People who drink one or two glasses of wine per day live longer and are less likely to die from all causes than either abstainers or heavy drinkers. Indeed, scientific researchers have found repeatedly that moderate daily wine consumption actually appears to be more beneficial than either zero consumption or over-consumption. A healthy lifestyle also includes regular exercise and a diet low in fat and high in fresh fruit, vegetables, and grains [45]. Consider muscadine wines for their medicinal value as well as their beverage value. Muscadine wines are made from the smarter grapes! Winemakers and wine lovers are fond of the saying:

"Per Vitem! Ad Vitam!"

The toast translates "Through the vine! To life!" according to the Knights of the Vine, which is a society that encourages the cultivation and use of vines and wines for good health.

The 2005 Dietary Guidelines for Americans, the official United States nutrition policy, advises, "If you drink alcoholic beverages, do so in moderation, with meals, and when consumption does not put you or others at risk." The Dietary Guidelines define moderation as "no more than one drink per day for women and no more than two drinks per day for men." For those adults who include wine in their lifestyle, it is useful to follow three simple rules:

1. Wine should be consumed only in moderation, and preferably around mealtime (as is done with Mediterranean cuisine).

2. Wine consumption should be part of social, family, celebratory or other occasions, but not as their central focus.

3. Excessive consumption should be discouraged, and the choice of abstinance for religious, health or personal reasons must be respected.

Total Phenolic Content of Muscadine Products- Along with the ORAC, FRAP or TEAC values that measure total antioxidant capacity of muscadine grapes, juices and other products, it is important to know what part is due to total phenolics and what is due to Vitamin C. Many scientists think that the disease-fighting benefits of fruits and berries is not just due to their ability to provide antioxidant protection. It is also very likely that phenolic compounds like resveratrol and quercetin produce specific responses such as reducing inflammation and improving health of the heart and other organs.

Guide to Muscadine Medicinal Chemistry - The words that describe phytochemicals of medicinal value are not familiar to most people. Therefore, we have provided definitions that may be helpful to non-chemists. Ellagic acid and ellagitannins are higher in muscadine grapes than in European wine grapes and Concord grapes. For a greater understanding of the classifications, structures, sources and biological properties of phytochemicals, there are many excellent books about natural products (pharmacognosy) [46, 47]

> **Anthocyanins and anthocyanidins**
> **Flavonols**
> **Flavanones**
> **Flavanols**
> **Flavones**
> **Stilbenes**
> **Ellagic acid and the Hydrolyzable Tannins**
> **Proanthocyanidins and the Condensed Tannins**

Of these classes, **muscadines are rich sources of anthocyanins, flavanols, flavonols and ellagic acid.** There is a large biomedical research literature supporting the health benefits of these classifications of bioflavonoids.

Phytochemicals- Chemicals manufactured by plants. In this book we are presenting some of the phytochemicals in muscadine grapes that are medicinally active when humans or companion animals consume them. Many pharmaceuticals are derived from plant substances, so the idea that they promote good health is not a new concept.

Bioflavonoids- A very large classification of compounds manufactured by living plants. These substances are polyphenolic compounds and there are thousands of them in the plant kingdom.

Flavonoids-Phytochemicals that contain a flavone ring (see Figure 3.4 and Table 3.1). Oftentimes, the word flavonoids is used when the reader knows that the compounds under discussion are the natural bioflavonoids. Natural bioflavonoids are phytochemicals.

Phenolics- Oftentimes, all substances with a phenolic ring are refered to as phenolics. In the nutraceutical industry, the phenolic content of a plant, its extracts or products, is used as a measure of the likely concentration of phenolic substances of medicinal value in the product. The test used to measure phenolics measures every compound with a phenolic ring. Flavonoids will be among the compounds included in this measurement. Plant phenolics represent a very large number of compounds that plants use for defensive purposes.

Polyphenolics is a term that refers to general structures of molecules that have two or more phenolic rings in the structure. Flavonoids and bioflavonoids are polyphenolic compounds. All of the categories shown above are polyphenolics, which are among the compounds measured in the ORAC test and the assay for Total Phenolics.

Catechins are monomeric flavanols (flavan-3-ols). Catechin and epicatechin exist in muscadines. Also, catechins are used as building blocks in proanthocyanidins (also called condensed tannins). Several (polymers) or many of these catechin units link together to form large molecules that are called oligomeric proanthocyanidins (OPCs). These large molecules exist in the seeds of the muscadine. Smaller units also exist in other fractions.

Anthocyanidins are the aglycones (no sugar molecule attached) of the corresponding anthocyanins. Examples of anthocyanidins in muscadines are cyanidin, delphinidin, peonidin, petunidin and malvidin.

Anthocyanins are cyanidins with a sugar molecule attached. Nature likes to attach sugar molecules to the anthocyanidins. An example is the cyanidin 3-O-glucoside. In this case glucose is attached.

Proanthocyanidins molecules built up using catechin units to make dimers and trimers (2 and 3 units) that are linked together.

Oligomeric Proanthocyanidins (OPCs) are 3 or more proanthocyanidins linked together. Some experts would classify any proanthocyanidins with more than 10 units as polymeric proanthocyanidins and would not include them in the OPC's.

Stilbenes are also defense molecules called alexins. The stilbene compounds (Figure 3.3) are synthesized by the plant for defense against pathogens, UV radiation, and other stresses. Muscadines have a family of stilbenes derived from resveratrol. Defense compounds are also called phytoalexins. One interesting theory about why resveratrol is protective in humans and animals is that our genes respond to plant defensive chemicals in a beneficial way.

Relationships Among Phytochemicals in Muscadines-

Within the plant, there are enzymes that convert one compound into another compound. The difficulty in understanding the chemistry arises because the names of the compounds sound so different that the relationships between these chemicals are not clear. Below is a highly simplified chart to illustrate the relationships between many of the compounds found in muscadines.

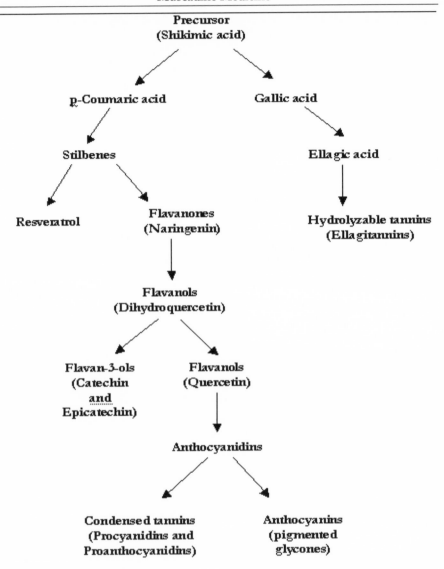

Figure 3.3. Pathways used to build up polyphenolics from simple building blocks. The building blocks have only one ring. As the compounds are built up, the structures become more complex. Some of the structures of phytochemicals in muscadine grapes are shown in Table 3.1.

Table 3.1. Names and Structures of Phytochemicals in Muscadine Grapes.

Class & Examples	Structure
One phenolic ring: Cinnamic acids Coumaric acid (shown), caffeic, ferulic, and chlorogenic acids	
One phenolic ring: Benzoic acids Gallic acid (shown), vanillic acid and protocatechuic acid	
Two phenolic rings: Stilbenes: Resveratrol, piceatannol and their glycosides	
Three rings (2 phenolic) Flavonoids: Quercetin and its relatives-apigenin, kaempferol, myricetin, luteolin	

Understanding of the Medicinal Value of Flavonoids-

Flavonoids are a large family of chemically related compounds synthesized by plants. Many of the substances that give plants color and taste are flavonoids. Because of their chemistry, they are excellent antioxidants. Plants use these substances for a variety of purposes. Of importance to the consumer is that flavonoids are now known to be bioactive in humans that consume them. In fact, this broad category of compounds probably accounts for many of the health benefits of high intakes of highly colored fruits and vegetables. Flavonoids that are known to be in muscadines include: cyanidin, delphinidin, malvidin, peonidin, petunidin, catechin, epicatechin, proanthocyanidins, quercetin, kaempferol, and myricetin.

Table 3.1 (continued)

Three rings: **Catechins** and their relatives: Epicatechin, epigallocatechin and epigallocatechin gallate (EGCG)	
Three rings: **Anthocyanins** are phenolics with no sugar. **Anthocyanidins** are glycated: Cyanidin, delphinidin, malvidin, pelargonidin, peonidin, petunidin	
Oligomeric **Procyanidins** or OPCs are formed from 2 or more anthocyanins by cross-linking the rings. Polymeric forms are called condensed tannins.	
Complex rings: Ellagic acid (top) and ellagitannins (bottom), which are hydrolyzable tannins built up from gallic acid. Ellagic acid has anti-cancer properties and is found in muscadines but not in European wine grapes.	

Absorption and Metabolism of Phytochemicals in Muscadines- Dietary substances need to get to the site of action to interact with biochemical processes. If the site of action is in the gastrointestinal tract, substances do not have to be absorbed. If substances act elsewhere, they need to be absorbed. While non-absorbed substances can exert actions via the inside of the gastrointestinal (GI) tract, many absorbed substances can also act on the GI tract when they are delivered back to the wall of the GI tract via the bloodstream. The GI tract has a very rich supply of blood. For other organs of the body, absorption of dietary substances is always an issue for scientists. We'll discuss two broad categories in muscadines. Because of the biomedical interest in these categories of compounds, there is a lot of analytical expertise being developed to follow the substances into the body, to identify the metabolites of the substances and finally, to identify how the body gets rid of the substances. There is more unknown than known. Let's review what is known to date and look forward to future information.

Absorption of flavonoids occurs mainly in the small intestine [48, 49]. In general flavonoids reach the small intestine in the same form they were in as they were ingested in the food. Most flavonoids appear in plants and foods as glycosides, meaning they have a sugar unit attached to their basic structure. These glycosides are stable to cooking temperatures, stomach acidity, and are not affected by stomach enzymes. Some flavonoids in natural products and in food supplements do not have a sugar molecule attached. These are called aglycones. Examples in muscadines are quercetin and kaempferol. A small fraction of these aglycones can be absorbed in the stomach, but most are absorbed in the small intestine.

Enzymes called hydrolases exist within the lumen, the brush border and within the cells lining the intestine [50]. These enzymes remove the sugar units from the flavonoids. Then, enzymes within the cells lining the intestine attach other molecules to the flavonoids in a process called conjugation. Conjugated flavonoids are now in a form that they can be transported into the blood stream. Most of these flavonoids are conjugated to glucuronic acid and are therefore referred to as glucuronides.

Following the glucuronidation reactions that take place during absorption, some of the flavonoids are metabolized further [52]. The liver can remove the glucuronide residue and replace it with a sulfate. This process is called sulfation. Another mechanism can then add a methyl group to another portion of the molecules. Flavonoids can be altered by the body and appear in different forms. An example is that quercetin can be taken in as just plain quercetin, but can appear in blood as quercetin, quercetin-3-glucuronide, quercetin-3'-sulfate, and methylquercetin-3-glucoronide [51] The free flavonoid and sulfate conjugates can be taken up by body tissues from the bloodstream by passive or facilitated diffusion mechanisms. Glucuronidated flavonoids are also taken up by body cells, but they have to be transported actively because they are more hydrophilic than the aglycone molecules. Once inside cells, these substances can be deconjugated and released as the basic flavonoid to interact with cellular mechanisms.

Excretion of Flavonoids- Some flavonoids are excreted via the kidney as glucuronides. While the percentage differs from flavonoid to flavonoid, the renal route of elimination is relatively small compared with the biliary/fecal route. Biliary secretion is the major route of excretion for flavonoids. The bile contains mostly glucoronidated and sulfated flavonoids. When the bile is secreted into the intestine, these conjugates move along with the intestinal contents and reach the ileum and colon. In the colon these conjugates are acted upon by microflora that naturally live in the colon. These bacteria then strip off the conjugated groups again and the free flavonoids are either further broken down by the bacteria or are available to get partially reabsorbed by the lining of the colon.

Absorption of Anthocyanins- Anthocyanins are flavonoids that are responsible for the colors blue, purple and red in grapes, berries, and various plants. They are most concentrated in deeply colored berries. In the US, average consumption is about 200 mg/day and is higher in summer when fresh berries and fruits are available [50]. Maximum consumption in the natural diet can easily exceed a gram a day because one cup of blueberries contains this much. Potential benefits include protection of blood vessels, vision, and nerve function. Because less than 1% of anthocyanins are absorbed, it seems likely that cells in which they are protective must concentrate the anthocyanins or one of their derivatives [52, 53]. This is not unusual. It is well known that carotenoids protect eyesight because certain cells in the macula accumulate them even though absorption is low and quite variable among individuals. For example, the carotenoid called lutein accumulates in the eye with a dietary intake of only 10 mg/day [54]. It is known that cells in the walls of blood vessels can accumulate anthocyanins [55].

Anthocyanins in fruits exist as aglycones and in many glycoside forms [50]. This is also true in muscadines [43, 56]. Muscadines contain cyanidin, delphinidin, peonidin, petunidin, malvidin [57]. Deep purple muscadines will have the highest levels of anthocyanins. Anthocyanins can be absorbed in the form of glycosides, but the percentage of anthocyanins absorbed is lower than for many other flavonoids. Plasma levels measured in human studies indicate low plasma levels in the nmol/L range after ingestion of known anthocyanin doses in the mg/kg range[58-62] Research is following anthocyanins from absorption to excretion. These substances have frustrated any number of scientists because either we do not know in what form to look for them or our ability to detect them is limited for technical reasons at the present time. An example is a study in which 6 women were given 189 g of blueberries that were analyzed to contain 690 mg of anthocyanins [58]. Amazingly, 5-8 different anthocyanins could be detected in urine samples during the first 6 hrs after the dose of blueberries, but levels of these anthocyanins were below the level of detection in plasma samples. The amount excreted in urine was only 0.004% of that in the dose. A somewhat higher 0.11%, but still very low urinary excretion rate, was observed by when the dose was from black currants[62]. It is currently estimated that perhaps 50% of anthocyanins stay in the gut and are never absorbed. This fraction has very beneficial effects on the gastrointestinal tract. While the amount or form of the absorbed anthocyanins is still frustrating the scientists, it is known that anthocyanins have profoundly beneficial health effects. Their whole story still needs to be revealed.

Health Benefits of Flavonoids- In general, flavonoids are good antioxidants. The plants that make them use them for antioxidant protection. Within the body, the flavonoids are also antioxidant. First, these substances can directly quench oxidative free radicals. Second, flavonoids can chelate metal ions that are often the catalysts for production of free radicals. Once chelated, the free metal ion is out of commission. Chelation mechanisms can decrease the oxidative stress of free iron and copper ions.

Flavonoids have more profound effects within the human body than can be explained by simple antioxidant or chelation activity. It is now known that these plant substances are helping cells to regulate gene expression in very beneficial ways. One way to look at chronic disease states like atherosclerosis, cancer, diabetes, or inflammatory and degenerative diseases is that they involve chronically adverse patterns of gene expression. As biologists have studied complex pathways involved in controlling the signals for regulating gene expression, it has become more and more obvious that phytochemicals in the diet play a major role in modulating these control systems. Flavonoids are not nutrients, not vitamins, not building blocks like essential amino acids or fatty acids. Yet, these so-called non-nutrients are powerful regulators of healthy gene expression patterns.

Some of the signalling pathways that can be modulated by flavonoids can control growth, proliferation and death of cancer cells. Others can modulate gene expression for mediators of inflammation. Still other actions of the flavonoids are that they can increase the activity of detoxification enzymes, inhibit platelet aggregation, increase arterial relaxation and decrease the expression of molecules on endothelial cells that line the blood vessel. This decreases the ability of the immune cells to move into the walls of arteries to produce an inflammatory focus that builds atherosclerotic plaques.

Disease Prevention by Flavonoids- While we'll discuss individual compounds below, patterns emerge from epidemiological data that diets highly enriched with flavonoids are protective against coronary heart disease, atherosclerosis in other arteries, cancer, neurodegenerative diseases and inflammatory diseases in general. A very good discussion of all the various studies can be found on the following website from the Linus Pauling Institute (see Web Resources). Muscadines make an excellent contribution to a disease prevention diet strategy.

Health Benefits of Anthocyanins- Anthocyanins in general are excellent antioxidants in a variety of test systems both in vitro and in vivo (For a review, see [50]). Even though absorption appears low, these substances are highly protective against oxidative stresses in a variety of animal models in the 1-2 mg/kg dose range. Anthocyanins are known to protect blood vessels in humans. These effects include antiedema and antioxidant effects that relate to blood vessel integrity. Fruits rich in anthocyanins have been thought for years to be highly protective of blood vessels in the eye and can improve night vision. Muscadines are rich in anthocyanins and proanthocyanins.

Antioxidant Properties of the Total Phenolic Fraction- It is important to understand that antioxidant properties of phenolics in fruits and vegetables contribute significantly to the health benefits of these compounds. First they quench free radicals and prevent the oxidation of important macromolecules that are essential for cellular functions. Second, they can regulate redox-sensitive systems in the body. Some of these are enzyme systems while others are systems that control gene expression. Others are involved in preventing oxidation of the cholesterol carrying particles in blood called LDL-cholesterol. While oxidation of body constituents is associated with aging of cells, antioxidants are considered to be anti-aging. Oxidative stress is a major component of chronic disease states. It is thought that oxidative processes contribute to the development of the disease state and fully participate in the maintenance of the disease.

How Extensive is the Biomedical Evidence for the Health Benefits of Single Phytochemicals Like Ellagic Acid and Resveratrol?- These are just two of the phytochemicals in muscadines with extensive biomedical documentation for their health benefits. For this book, we have searched the literature on every substance of biomedical interest in muscadines. We'd like the reader to know how to do this and judge for themselves. Too often, persons who are non-scientists turn to Internet websites that may or may not have valid information. It is always possible to look up the full biomedical literature to judge validity of website information. Authoritative websites will usually cite the primary biomedical literature. Here is how to search the primary literature.

How To Find Biomedical Literature Concerning Muscadine Chemicals- If the reader searches the biomedical literature, he or she will find that more research has been published. Just type www.pubmed.gov in the browser. Look at the search box at the top and type in one of the following phenolic compounds. The reader will see a discrepancy between the number of papers below and the number at the time of reading this text. This field is expanding rapidly. By the time this book is published, there will be more references than we cited. The reader should remain vigilant. The writers promise to update this book regularly in future additions to keep abreast of the health potential of muscadine products. One can narrow the subject area of the search by typing in specific subject areas. For example:

Ellagic Acid (Total refs = 628)

Ellagic Acid and Cancer = 113 refs

Ellagic Acid and Chemoprevention = 22 refs

Ellagic Acid and Antioxidant = 118 refs

Ellagic Acid and Cardiovascular = 23 refs

Ellagic Acid and Diabetes = 4 refs

Ellagic Acid and Gene Expression = 6

Ellagic Acid and Aldose Reductase Inhibition = 7

Ellagic Acid and Inflammation = 8

Resveratrol (Total refs = 1081)

Resveratrol and Cancer = 371 refs

Resveratrol and Chemoprevention = 47 refs

Resveratrol and Antioxidant = 831 refs

Resveratrol and Anti-aging = 23

Resveratrol and Cardiovascular = 131

Resveratrol and Diabetes = 2

Resveratrol and Gene Expression = 109

Resveratrol and Inflammation = 31

Resveratrol and Brain = 46

Chlorogenic Acid (Total refs = 744)

Chlorogenic Acid and Cancer = 44 refs

Chlorogenic Acid and Chemoprevention = 6 refs

Chlorogenic Acid and Antioxidant = 226 refs

Chlorogenic Acid and Anti-aging = 2 refs

Chlorogenic Acid and Cardiovascular = 23 refs

Chlorogenic Acid and Diabetes = 12 refs

Chlorogenic Acid and Gene Expression = 16 refs

Chlorogenic Acid and Inflammation = 4 refs

Chlorogenic Acid and Brain = 9 refs

Chlorogenic Acid and Immune System = 24 refs

Chlorogenic Acid and Gastrointestinal System

Esophagus = 1 ref; Gastric = 9 refs; Small Intestine = 7 refs;

Colon = 14 refs; epithelial cells in general = 10 refs

Similarly, the reader can verify the number of research papers for other phytochemicals in muscadine. Here is what we found:

Caffeic Acid = 1203 refs

Cinnamic Acid = 560 refs

Catechin = 2817 refs

Epicatechin = 2645 refs

Gallic Acid = 2996 refs

Geraniol = 370 refs

p-Coumaric Acid = 382 refs

Kaempferol = 959 refs

Myricetin = 350 refs

Quercetin = 4086 refs

Tartaric Acid = 727 refs

Cyanidin = 283 refs

Peonidin = 73 refs

Delphinidin = 133 refs

Petunidin = 44 refs

Malvidin = 108 refs

Pectin = 2359 refs

Vitamin C = 29,606

Derivatives of Phytochemicals have Bioactivities Too! The list above looks very short. It is actually the tip of the iceberg because each of these substances gives rise to a myriad of derivative substances within the plant and then again inside the human body. Each of the derivative substances may have their own profile of bioactivities. This can be greater than, or less than or simply different than the parent compound. Let us take resveratrol for example and look at it and its derivatives that are bioactive. Unless the analytical lab is set up to analyze all its derivatives, only the actual resveratrol is assayed. This may seriously underestimate the presence of this substance. This oftentimes accounts for ranges of resveratrol levels from undetectable to the 450 ppm range. The plant has the ability to park resveratrol as some derivative products.

Example: Resveratrol and Its Close Cousins- Resveratrol is one product in a biochemical pathway in plants called the phenylpropanoid pathway. Most of the substances in this pathway have biomedical activities. Resveratrol is 3,4,5'-

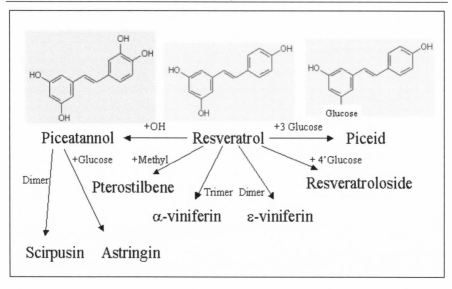

Figure 3.4. Resveratrol is converted to other stilbenes such as piceid and piceatannol that have important health benefits in humans.

trihydroxystilbene. It is synthesized from 4 Coumaryl CoA + 3 Malonyl CoAs. It is important to realize that this phenylpropanoid pathway is activated in the plant by stress, including UV radiation and fungal attacks. Resveratrol is a good anti-fungal compound for the plant to put in its skin to prevent invasion by fungi. This includes yeasts. Muscadines have this pathway and it is probably highly active because of the hot, humid and brutally sunny weather the grapes get exposed to in the SE USA. In looking at the figure below, it is obvious that resveratrol is not the end of the line. It is the basic structure for multiple other resveratrol-like compounds that can be produced to "park" resveratrol as endproducts and still keep the pathways flowing. These metabolites are active endproducts and may contribute much more resveratrol-like activity than the amount of resveratrol that can be measured in the product itself. For example, piceids have been shown to appear in red grape juices at concentrations 6-7 times higher than resveratrol itself[63] and also appears in red wines[64] This can be a big advantage to anyone ingesting these juices because at least two groups have reported that some phenolic substances are better absorbed from the gastrointestinal tract if they have are conjugated to a glucose (glucosides). [65, 66]. The piceids are glucosides of resveratrol and may enhance the amount of resveratrol that gets into the bloodstream. In some grape juices, there may be 10X more piceids than resveratrol [63]. If this is true in the juice and the wines, it is obviously also true in the skins and seeds. Similarly, the other "resveratrol-like" compounds need to be analyzed to understand the total nutraceutical contribution of this family of compounds. Each are extremely bioactive and contribute to the nutraceutical potential of the products. Confusion arises in the literature when only "resveratrol" is analyzed. Greater work, instrumentation and expense is necessary to obtain a full spectrum of the resveratrol family. Most analytical labs are not set up to do this, but they will be in the future as the biomedical interest in these compounds grows.

In the case of piceid, the glucose unit is attached at position 3. If glucose is attached to position 4, the compound is called resveratroloside. Similarly, a methyl group can be attached to produce pterostilbene; a dehydroxylation can produce piceatannol that can in turn have a glucose attached to become astringin. There is yet another way that resveratrol can be stored efficiently. Two molecules of it can combine and form ε-viniferin and if there are three molecules condensing into one, it is called α-viniferin. Similarly, if two molecules of piceatannol condense, they form a new molecule called scirpusin.

The analogues of resveratrol may be as active or even more active than resveratrol itself. One recent study tested the potency of pterostilbene, resveratrol, piceatannol and resveratrol trimethyl ether against the known effect of a cholesterol-lowering drug, ciprofibrate. The test results indicated that pterostilbene, but not resveratrol, was an excellent activator of PPARα. In fact, it was better than the drug ciprofibrate [67]. It also was much more potent than resveratrol and the other two analogs. Pterostilbene was then tested for its cholesterol-lowering ability in the hypercholesterolemic hamster. This animal model is used to test many drugs that lower cholesterol. Pterostilbene at 25 ppm in diet reduced LDL cholesterol 29%, raised HDL cholesterol 7% and lowered blood glucose by 14%[70]. All of these are beneficial effects.

Additivity and Synergism Among Phytochemicals Is the whole equal to the sum or its parts or more than the sum of its parts? Above we have given you the current list of bioactive substances in the phenolic fraction of the muscadine and the overwhelming number of studies that are forming the biomedical literature for each of them. We will attempt to derive the most important properties of each of these compounds from this literature. We will discuss it in terms the non-scientist can understand. Next, we will make a case for how these chemicals can act synergistically (more than the sum of the parts). Finally, we will discuss work that has been done on muscadines. The health benefits of muscadines may be the best kept secret of the South.

Self Care and Maximal Health- In Western society, the body is often times treated like a machine. If a part in an automobile breaks down, it gets fixed or replaced. By analogy, if a body part breaks down, we go to someone who specializes in fixing that body part. The problem is that the body is more like a garden than a machine. It needs to be nurtured and cared for daily. As nutrition science has become more evolved, it is embracing information from other scientific disciplines to fully understand how to best nurture the body by dietary intake each day. We now speak in new terms that reflect major advances in the sciences. The human genome has been sequenced. Now, functional genomics is the challenge of the present. Nutrient control of gene expression and signaling pathways are very important areas of nutrition science. Nutraceutical science is also a new concept. It involves using knowledge of both modern nutrition science and modern pharmacology to produce products that have beneficial effects within the living system. In this book, we emphasize the phytochemicals in muscadines and the effect these chemicals have within the living system. The upsurge of interest in flavonoids and tannins and other phenolics and polyphenolics has been explosive. Our understanding of the health benefits of a high vegetable and fruit intake is boiling down to understanding the roles of phytochemicals in controlling various processes in the body. In past years, these phytochemicals were ignored by most health researchers. Today, we have national health advocacy agencies making dietary recommendations for health maintenance and disease prevention based upon phytochemicals in dietary choices for a prevention diet. We hope that by the end of this book that we have given the reader ample reasons to understand how choices in diet can influence risk for chronic disease states. We put forward the muscadine grape as a wonderful and powerful nutraceutical choice to include in that 21st Century diet.

Multivitamins now contain some phytochemicals, but don't look for that timy multivitamin tablet to contain the spectrum and holistic balance of phytochemicals that one can get in whole fruits and vegetables. Natural balances of phytochemicals can also be obtained in food supplement and nutraceutical products. Powders of fruit skins and fruit seeds or whole fruits are manufactured to retain the phytochemicals while removing the water. Extracts usually draw out a desired fraction of phytochemicals and leave behind the water and fiber and other chemical fractions. The products are still balanced because they contain a natural spectrum of the plant's phytochemicals

Diets vary in phytochemical content. It is clear that a natural diet contains at least 100 mg and certainly up to 1000 mg (1 gram) of phytochemicals per day. We believe that evidence-based medical research is consistent with a path to improved health based on a plan to take in 100-1000 mg of phytochemicals each day. When fresh produce such as muscadine grapes is not available in the market, it is reasonable to consider an enriched supplement such as powdered grape skins and/or seeds (pomace) as part of your own self-care regimen.

Finally, we do not believe that taking pills with purified chemicals is the preferred path to achieving a healthy diet. The body prefers balance, not imbalance. A food supplement containing grape skins or grape seeds is actually a very complex mixture of hundreds of chemicals. These are highly balanced products, not purified substances. Similarly, extracts of these fractions contain many different compounds. Again, they are a highly balanced mixture of substances that is enriched in a certain profile by extraction. Natural balance is maintained within the context of using it as a food supplement within the rest of the diet. We don't believe that the same beneficial effects are attainable by purifying just one plant molecule and taking it in a highly concentrated form that acts as a "drug". Taking the natural mixtures of phytochemicals in plants is a natural medicine and nutritional approach to health maintenance and disease prevention. The goal is to achieve and maintain balance by taking in a well-balanced nutritional milieu. This is not alternative medicine. This is complementary medicine. It can easily be integrated into any plan that requires drug therapy. We argue that integrative medicine is the best approach to health problems. Food supplements and nutraceuticals and vitamins and minerals are logical products to replenish modern diets that have veered too far away from whole foods. With proper diet selections, one can minimize the number of food supplements needed.

Web Resources

Clinical Trials.gov: http://www.clinicaltrials.gov

Entrez-PubMed home page for PubMed search: http://www.pubmed.gov

North Carolina Winery muscadine web page:
http://www.ncwine.org/muscadine/muscadineHealth.html

Knights of the Vine, http://www.kov-dc.org/

U.S. Patent and Trademark Office patent database: http://www.uspto.gov/

Linus Pauling Institute, a national center for the study of complementary and alternative medicine. http://lpi.oregonstate.edu/

National Center for Complementary and Alternative Medicine (a branch of the National Institutes of Health): http://nccam.nih.gov/

Office of Dietary Supplements (a unit in the National Institutes of Health that provides current information about supplements): http://ods.od.nih.gov/

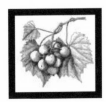

Chapter 4-

Muscadines vs. Heart Disease and Cholesterol

Dietary protection against heart disease is generally designed to provide both antioxidant and anti-inflammatory support for blood vessel health. It also supports heart muscle health, blood pressure control, healthy blood lipid profiles, anti-coagulation and good blood glucose control. Heart disease is most often coronary heart disease, a disease of the blood vessels that supply the heart muscle with oxygen and nutrients. Atherosclerotic plaque buildup in the coronary arteries occurs with time until it partially occludes the blood vessels. Heart attacks occur (myocardial infarcts) when a partially occluded coronary artery is rapidly plugged up with a blood clot and possibly blood vessel constriction at the site of an atherosclerotic plaque or a series of plaques. While the myocardial infarction is a rapid event, it occurs very late in the coronary artery disease sequence. Since building atherosclerotic plaques takes years, avoiding atherosclerosis can be accomplished with early choice of diets that are anti-atherosclerotic and staying with those diets throughout adult life

Reduction of Oxidative Stress Damage to the Cardiovascular System-

The key is to alter the microenvironment throughout the vascular system and make endothelial cells healthy. Endothelial cell dysfunction occurs in many disease states and conditions that accelerate atherosclerosis and cardiovascular disease [71-76]. Dietary polyphenols confer protection to the cardiovascular system in multiple ways over and above their high antioxidant protection [68].

The diagram below shows how two species of oxidative stressors are elevated in multiple conditions. Hypertension, diabetes, smoking, elevated LDL, elevated homocysteine levels and estrogen deficiency are some of the factors that can exert oxidative stress on endothelial cells and vascular smooth muscles cells. Flavonoids and other polyphenolics have been shown to be helpful in each of these conditions. In smoking, the best solution is to stop immediately. Phytochemicals can do a lot to improve the oxidative stress state due to smoking. Of course, continued smoking will work against antioxidant progress.

When stressed vascular endothelial cells are in high oxidative disease states, they first "activate" and then start to dysfunction[69-76]. This leads to cell death (apoptosis), leukocyte adhesion (telling immune cells to invade here), lipid deposition (more cholesterol deposited to build the plaque), vasoconstriction (muscle contracts and narrows vessel), vascular smooth muscle growth

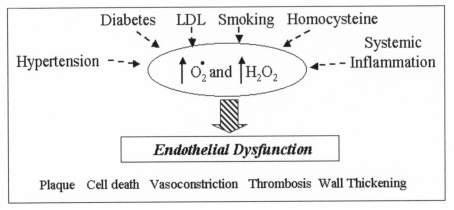

Figure 4.1. Blood vessels become unhealthy in diabetes partly because increased production of reactive oxygen species such as superoxide and hydrogen peroxide contributes to tissue damage.

and thrombosis (blood clot). Phytochemicals within muscadines fight each of these processes. One clue is that the phenolic substances within muscadines are more powerful than vitamin E or the carotenoids as antioxidants. Dietary consumption of flavonoids has been shown to be inversely related to morbidity and mortality from coronary heart disease [77-80] Muscadines are high in flavonoids, anthocyanins, OPCs and hydrolyzable tannins (polymers of ellagic and gallic acid). Each of these groups is potent antioxidants that contribute to protection of the vascular endothelial cells. Juice and wine contain high concentrations of these substances. This helps explains why moderate wine consumption has proved beneficial to the cardiovascular system[81-83].

Inhibition of LDL Oxidation- The protective role of phytochemicals is often demonstrated by their ability to inhibit oxidation of LDL-cholesterol. LDL stands for low-density lipoprotein. LDL is a particle in blood that carries cholesterol. It is sometimes referred to as "bad cholesterol" because its elevation in blood is thought to contribute to the atherosclerotic process. LDL particles can be oxidized to oxidized-LDL particles under conditions associated with oxidative stress (like diabetes, metabolic syndrome, hypertension, high fat, high calorie diets). The oxidized-LDL is the real "bad cholesterol" because it can be used more readily for building atherosclerotic plaques and it is also toxic to the vascular endothelial cell and activates macrophages. Macrophages are immune cells that help build atheroslerotic plaques by ingesting LDL.

Oxidation of LDL involves oxidation of many of its consitutents molecules, including its apolipoproteins B-100, phospholipids, fatty acids and cholesterol. During oxidative attack, the first thing that happens is that the LDL particles antioxidant protections in consumed. Vitamin E and carotenoids are present within LDL to protect it from oxidation. After they are oxidized, polyunsaturated fatty acids and cholesterol become susceptible to attack. Cholesterol is oxidized to oxysterols [84]. Polyunsaturated fatty acids like arachidonic acid are oxidized to isoprostanes and epoxyisoprostanes[85]. When the apolipoprotein B-100 is modified by oxidation, it can no longer bind to LDL receptors to remove cholesterol from the bloodstream. At this time, the whole LDL particle is altered and becomes very attractive to macrophages, the immune system's scavengers of abnormal debris. The process of LDL oxidation occurs more readily in the artery wall at a focus building an atherosclerotic plaque.

Polyphenolic Inhibition of LDL Oxidation- Scientists can set up a laboratory test system with LDL to measure the ability of various substances to inhibit the oxidation of LDL to ox-LDL. The flavanol, flavonol, anthocyanidin, OPC and tannin substances in muscadines are powerful inhibitors of LDL oxidation. Using such systems, catechins [86], quercetin, kaempferol [87] caffeic acid and p-coumaric acids [88] have been shown to inhibit oxidation of LDL.

There is a direct relationship between the total polyphenolic content of fruit juices and wines and their ability to inhibit oxidation of LDL. Example, red wine high in polyphenolics was many times better at inhibiting formation of ox-LDL than white wine, that is lower in total polyphenols. This is true for muscadine wines also. The red wines are higher in total phenolics than the white wines. Muscadine skins and seeds are extremely high in total phenolic compound content and their antioxidant capacity is very high. It is easy to understand how eating a daily diet high in antioxidants can inhibit ox-LDL formation and lower the rate of atherosclerosis. Indeed, the relationship between diet and atherosclerosis is widely accepted.

Endothelial Cell Health is Paramount- Protection and good function of the blood vessel is largely dependent on good endothelial cell function. Vascular endothelial cells are the important cells that line the blood vessels. These cells interact directly with substances in the blood and also send signals to smooth muscle cells and connective tissue cells that compose the major part of the blood vessel wall. Endothelial cell health is important for regulating blood pressure, maintaining proper blood clotting and impeding the development of atherosclerotic plaques. In other words, maintaining healthy endothelial cells is in large measure the key to avoiding coronary artery disease and strokes. Purple grape juice has been shown to improve endothelial function while reducing the susceptibiliity of LDL to oxidation in patients[89, 90].

Atherosclerosis as an Inflammatory Disease Atherosclerosis is known to be an inflammatory disease. Inflammatory diseases are characterized by a high degree of oxidative stress that leads to damage of healthy tissues. Both the inflammation process and the oxidative stress process lead to an "activation" of the vascular endothelial cell. This "activation" accelerates the rate of atheroslerosis. Ox-LDL is one factor that can lead to "activation" of the vascular endothelium. Nature designed this process of "activation" as a way for vascular endothelial cells to coax monocytes (white blood cells that are part of the immune system) to come to an area of infection or damage. In itself, this is a normal process involved in repair and healing of damaged or infected areas of the blood vessel wall.

Unfortunately, this process is chronically activated in many people and it leads to a condition called systemic inflammation. In this condition, there is generalized "activation" of vascular endothelial cells, high oxidative stress and enhanced invasion of the blood vessel walls by monocytes. Once these monocytes pass the endothelial lining of the blood vessels, they are called macrophages. Macrophages are programmed to ingest bacteria, cellular debris and love to ingest LDL particles in the walls of blood vessels. In fact, they seem to prefer ox-LDL particles[91]. They reside in the blood vessel wall and ingest so much ox-LDL that they are called foam cells because they actually look foamy under the microscope[92]. These foam cells are the mechanism by which cholesterol from LDL keeps building atherosclerotic plaques. These macrophages also change the activities of underlying smooth muscle cells in the vascular wall. Some muscle cells "become fibroblasts" and move into the atherosclerotic plaque. Their function is to lay down a lot of fiber and collagen that helps build the plaque. In the meantime, the endothelial cells keep trying to cover the plaque and keep everything smooth inside the blood vessel. With time, however, the bulging plaque causes the blood to exert so much shear stress on its contours that the endothelial covering is actually worn off and swept away. When this happens, all the components within the atherosclerotic plaque are exposed directly to the blood. Platelets are immediately activated and a clot starts to form. In addition, relaxing chemicals released by the endothelial cells are no longer present and there is an imbalance of chemicals being released that cause the blood vessel to constrict. **The situation of ruptured plaque + blood clot + vessel constriction in a coronary artery is what usually causes a heart attack.**

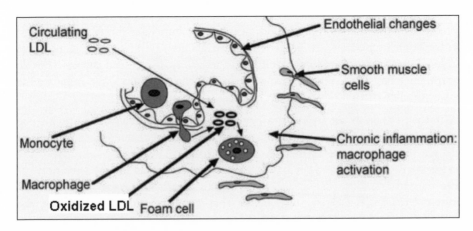

Figure 4.2. How LDL-cholesterol contributes to atherosclerosis and plaque formation in the wall of blood vessels.

Muscadine grapes have multiple phytochemicals that keep the endothelial cells healthy, keep LDL from becoming ox-LDL, decrease the movement of monocytes from the bloodstream, decrease inflammation, decrease "activation" of endothelial cells, decrease atherosclerotic plaque formation and overall decrease the risk of heart attacks in particular and atherosclerosis in general.

The same process that leads to a heart attack can also produce a stroke, which is why these are sometimes called brain attacks. Decreasing the rate of atherosclerosis can improve the health of any organ that has plaques building. For example, peripheral vascular disease is a major problem for circulation in the legs and feet.

Other Vascular Protective Functions of Polyphenols Besides protecting the vasculature and LDL from oxidative attack, polyphenolic phytochemicals also enhance the production of vasodilating factors, specifically nitric oxide, endothelium-derived hyperpolarizing factor and prostacyclin[68]. Discussion of these systems would be lengthy and can be reviewed in [70].

Erectile Dysfunction A problem with endothelial cell dysfunction underlies many cases of male erectile dysfunction. If the endothelial cells of the blood vessels supplying blood to the corpus cavernosum are not able to produce enough nitric oxide erectile dysfunction results. The general ability of phytochemicals to support both the integrity of the endothelial cell and its nitric oxide signalling pathway is well known [93]. Protection of the endothelial cells in the entire vasculature is highly affected by a diet high in the polyphenolics in fruits and vegetables. Flavonoids, catechins, tannins and other polyphenolics like the OPCs are all thought to contribute [93]. Muscadine grape skins + grape seeds are high in these categories of compounds.

Recently, mixtures of grape skin anthocyanins (muscadines are very high in these) were found to have very good phosphodiesterase E5 inhibitors[94] in the phenolic fraction. The drugs sildenafil, vardenafil and tadalafil are pharmaceutical phosphodiesterase E5 inhibitors[95]. The reader will recognize these drugs under the tradenames **Viagra®, Levitra® and Cialis®**, respectively. In summary, the phenolics in grapes not only protect endothelial and vascular cells from oxidative damage, they also help blood vessel vasodilation. In the case of erectile dysfunction, polyphenolics can protect endothelial cells from damage in the first place, and can improve the nitric oxide signalling system by causing the upregulation of endothelial nitric oxide synthase and also by inhibiting PDE5. **Who'd-a-thunk muscadines would share an activity with Viagra®?** The take home message is that caring for blood vessels is good preventive medicine.

Cholesterol. We are bombarded with commercials concerning the need to lower cholesterol. These commercials are usually pharmaceutical ads for cholesterol-lowering drugs. We know that these drugs possess significant toxicities, either because we have read the package inserts at prescription time or we listen to the trailers mandated on the TV commericials concerning the side effects of these drugs. Because of these side effects and the fact that these are generally prescribed for chronic use, many people look toward cholesterol-lowering diet, food supplements and nutraceuticals for maintaining lower cholesterol.

Regardless of one's absolute total cholesterol, LDL level or LDL/HDL ratio or TG levels it is important to aim for HEALTHY CHOLESTEROL and HEALTHY TOTAL BLOOD LIPID PROFILES. People get heart attacks at any cholesterol level, (see Framingham heart statistics), so there is a lot more to preventing heart attacks than just cholesterol. As indicated above, keeping cholesterol from oxidizing is very important. A good strategy for maintaining or achieving healthy cholesterol is to eat a diet that tends to lower LDL cholesterol, keeps LDL from oxidizing and lowers triglycerides. GOOD NEWS! The same plant based diet containing 10-12 servings a day of deeply colored vegetables and fruit is the basis of a cholesterol-lowering, healthy blood lipid profile and anti-inflammatory diet. Parenthetically, it is also the basis of an anti-hypertensive, anti-cancer and anti-obesity diet. For additional power, concentrated forms of specific natural products are available in food supplements or in nutraceutical products to enhance the medicinal value of the plant-based diet recommended for overall health. These are convenient for people who cannot eat the full range of deeply colored vegetables and fruit daily. This doesn't mean that one needs to become a vegetarian. It just means that a small portion of meat or lowfat dairy can be eaten with a basic whole plant food diet. There are many high protein soy-based products and legume products that can help lower the amount of animal-based food in the modern diet.

Muscadines and Cholesterol. In addition to decreasing oxidation of LDL, the phytochemicals in muscadines may actually help lower cholesterol levels. There hasn't been very much work done on this to date, but we note that Dr. Betty Ector has described work she did with muscadines in rats. Dr. Ector reports that a powder of muscadine puree added to the diet of a rat given cholesterol and choline would significantly prevent the rise of serum total cholesterol, LDL cholesterol and triglycerides and liver triglycerides. In addition, she found that the muscadine puree powder was more effective in elevating serum HDL-cholesterol than oat bran [96]. Ellagitannins are inhibitors of squalene epoxidase, an enzyme that participates in cholesterol biosynthesis[97]. This could be another mechanism whereby cholesterol biosynthesis is affected by muscadines that are high in ellagitannins. Evidence is accumulating that suggests grape phytochemicals may help lower LDL, raise HDL and lower triglycerides [98].

Flavonoids are Cardioprotective Heart disease and stroke are both lower in groups of people who consume higher amounts of flavonoids in their diets [78, 99], and the risk of myocardial infarction is lower in people who consume quercetin, kaempferol and myricetin in foods and beverages [100]. These are the main flavonols found in muscadine grapes. Diets that contain higher levels of flavonols are correlated with lower levels of LDL-cholesterol [101].

Quercetin Protects Blood Vessels Flavonols seem to protect the heart by affecting the blood vessel wall, the blood clotting system, and the heart itself. Quercetin relaxes the blood vessel wall [102], and a relaxed wall improves blood flow and prevents clotting. Quercetin and resveratrol both increase the production of enzymes that dissolve blood clots (tissue plasminogen activator [103] and tissue factor [104]). Both flavonols also block production of an enzyme that contributes to atherosclerosis [105]. The enzyme is called inducible nitric oxide synthase, or iNOS, and it contributes to inflammation in the blood vessel wall.

Heart attacks often occur because blood clots form in the arteries of the heart. Quercetin and resveratrol both block the triggers to blood clotting such as the activation of thrombin [106] and platelet aggregation [107-109]. Blood clots deprive the heart of oxygen, but quercetin improves heart function when blood flow is reduced and protects against loss of the heart rhythm [110, 111]. If a person has elevated blood pressure, the heart tends to grow (ventricular hypertrophy), and quercetin may oppose this enlargement [112]. Therefore, evidence is growing that quercetin and other flavonols in muscadine grapes promote healthier levels of cholesterol, prevent blood clotting, protect the blood vessel wall, and defend the heart when it is deprived of oxygen.

Resveratrol and Cardiovascular Health The health benefits of resveratrol were first popularized as scientists looked for clues in explaining the "French Paradox". The question was why do French get away with eating all the high fat culinary delights, pastries and cheeses that we Americans are told produces heart attacks? The first hypothesis after analyzing diets was that the French drink a lot of red wine and drink it daily. Briefly, the daily ingestion of red wine was found to be statistically protective against atherosclerosis and heart attacks. Both the alcohol and the phenolic content of red wine, or and interaction between the two have been proposed to account for the "French Paradox"[113, 114]. Among the protective phenolics in red wine are resveratrol and its derivatives. These occur in higher concentrations in red wines because these wines are initially fermented with the pomace and the resveratrol compounds are extracted into the wine. Since the curiosity of the "French Paradox", a lot of work has shown that resveratrol does indeed have cardioprotective actions[115-117]. Atherosclerosis is now known to be an inflammatory disease of the blood vessel wall. In general, anti-inflammatory compounds tend to be protective against coronary artery disease, atherosclerosis and stroke. Resveratrol inhibits platelet aggregation [116, 118-120].Platelet aggregation is a major factor in precipitation of myocardial infarctions and strokes.

Resveratrol, Inhibition of NF-kappaB activation and Inhibition of Cell Adhesion Molecule Gene Expression- Resveratrol inhibits the gene expression for vascular and immune cell adhesion molecules[121-125]. These adhesion molecules get expressed in inflammation states and are used to recruit monocytes (white blood cells that become macrophages) into the inflamed region of the vessel wall. Neutophils also access the inflammation site using cell adhesion molecules[122]. In the blood vessel wall, the monocytes become macrophages and start to very aggressively ingest ox-LDL. This process builds the atherosclerotic plaque. Activation of NF-kappaB is highly involved in regulating scores of genes associated with inflammatory processes. Among these are the cell adhesion molecules and cytokines involved in the inflammatory process. Resveratrol is known to inhibit activation of NF-kappaB [126-137].

Resveratrol and eNOS expression- Another action that resveratrol has on vascular endothelial cells (cells that line all blood vessels) is to stimulate them to produce a vasodilator substance called nitric oxide (NO)[138-142]. NO is synthesized by an enzyme called eNOS (endothelial nitric oxide synthase). The action of NO on vascular smooth muscles is to get them to relax. A relaxation of vascular smooth muscle lowers blood pressure and enhances the function of various vasculatures around the body. Resveratrol and its analogues are among a host of polyphenolics in grapes and wine that have this effect on eNOS[142] Resveratrol stimulates eNOS activity. This is thought to be highly cardioprotective. Resveratrol inhibits proliferation of vascular smooth muscles cells that occurs underneath the atherosclerotic plaque[143-147].

Cardiovascular Protection is a Multifactorial Challenge As indicated above, the atherosclerotic process leading to heart disease and stroke is a very complex process. The process usually involves dyslipidemia, oxidative stress, inflammation, inflammatory cytokines, endothelial dysfunction, smoolth muscle cell proliferation and enhanced thrombus formation. **This means there are multiple mechanisms of intervention in order to arrest or reverse the process.** One area in which there is very good evidence for beneficial effects of grape phytochemicals in their ability to keep LDL from forming ox-LDL. In addition, there is an enormous literature accumulating to support a beneficial role of grape phytochemicals in heart and vascular health in general[90, 113, 114, 118, 119, 148-160]. Evidence for these effects comes from many animal model studies, cell culture studies, molecular biological and biochemical studies and human epidemiological and clinical studies.

We've received many reports from persons who take muscadine food supplements and nutraceuticals that their cholesterol levels are "way down". Now, scientists can't do anything with anecdotal acounts, but anecdotal accounts oftentimes encourage scientific inquiry. Work is ongoing in several laboratories to further study muscadine-specific grape seed, grape skin, grape pomace and extracts of these fractions for their ability to positively affect hypercholesterolemia (and other conditions) in animal models. Muscadines have an array of phytochemicals known to be highly protective of the cardiovascular system[90, 113, 114, 118, 119, 148-160].

Highlights of Muscadine Phytochemicals and Cardiovascular Health

1. Grape seed procyanidins (and other phytochemicals) improve atherosclerotic risk indices in rats, hamsters, rabbits[23, 149-151, 156, 161-165].

2. Grape phytochemicals help keep cholesterol healthy.   These phytochemicals should be part of any cholesterol-lowering effort. Grape seed decreases susceptibility of LDL-cholesterol to oxidation. Grape seed extracts have been shown to help protect the formation of Ox-LDL even in humans who smoke [166-168].

3. Grape seed phytochemicals have many cardioprotective actions[21, 169-171].

4. Grapes, grape juice, wines, grape skins and grape seeds have phytochemicals highly beneficial to endothelial cell functions and the cardiovascular system[172-180].

5. Grape seed phytochemicals affect macrophages beneficially[32, 36, 149, 181-183]. This is particularly important in atherosclerosis[149].

6. Grape seed phytochemicals are known to be highly anti-inflammatory in many experimental models [23, 184-187].

7. Grape seed and grape skin phytochemicals are highly antioxidant [43, 57, 188-196] and therefore highly protective in high oxidative stress states like hypertension.

8. Grape phytochemicals inhibit activation of NF-kappa B, a nuclear transcription factor that powerfully regulates gene expression involved in inflammatory responses and activation of the vascular endothelial cell [121, 179, 197-200].

9. Grape skin extracts have been shown to reduce blood pressure in two animal models of hypertension. Evidence suggested grape skin extract protected endothelium-dependent vasodilation[201].

10. Cumulative evidence indicates there are substances in muscadines have cholesterol-lowering properties. The stilbenes are among these substances[67, 155].

Medicinal Value of Muscadine Wines and Juices- Almost everyone knows about the "French wine paradox," which is the idea that people in France eat a lot of fat but still have a low incidence of heart disease compared to the United States. It doesn't seem fair. There is debate about why this is the case, but most researchers believe it is due either to the phytochemicals in the wines, to the alcohol itself or to the combination [202-206].

At present, the benefits of muscadine wines have not specifically been studied regarding heart disease, but the prediction is that they would also protect against heart disease. The reason is that the phytochemical content of muscadine grapes is similar (we think better) compared to that found in European grapes. The protective chemicals are polyphenols (flavonoids), and the muscadine has abundant polyphenols. These phytochemicals are easily dissolved in alcohol, so wine is essentially a way of delivering these substances to the body. Alcohol expands the blood vessels and improves circulation, especially to the heart after meals. Having a civilized glass of wine with a meal adds muscadine power to a diet that is healthy for the heart and blood vessels!

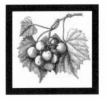

Chapter 5-

Muscadines vs. Prediabetes, Diabetes and Metabolic Syndrome

Two Kinds of Diabetes- Type I diabetes used to be called juvenile diabetes because it usually occurs in childhood. However, some adults also get Type I diabetes when the cells that make insulin are attacked by the immune system. The cells die and can no longer make insulin. In people with Type I diabetes, insulin needs to be taken for life and blood sugar needs to be regulated constantly with diet, exercise and medications. **Type II diabetes** used to be defined as the kind of diabetes people get when they are over 40, but increasingly pediatricians are finding it in children and teens. It was called adult onset diabetes or non-insulin dependent because people with this kind of diabetes are still making insulin, but they don't respond to it very well. This condition is called *insulin resistance*. There are many patterns and causes of Type II diabetes, but often it develops along with abdominal obesity. Suffice it to say that the Type II diabetics need to control blood sugar, reverse insulin resistance, avoid or reverse obesity and follow a very healthy diet plan to avoid a lifetime of drugs and diabetic complications. The incidence of Type II diabetes is rapidly increasing in the USA.   Obesity and metabolic syndrome predispose an individual toward developing Type II diabetes. Needless to say, both obesity and metabolic syndrome have also reached epidemic levels in the US.

Metabolic Syndrome- Metabolic syndrome (sometimes referred to as metabolic syndrome X) was identified by Dr. Gerald Reaven [207]. It is actually a cluster of interacting metabolic and vascular disorders (see Table 5.1). Characteristics of metabolic syndrome are impaired glucose tolerance, decreased insulin sensitivity, hyperglycemia, and a risk-prone blood lipid profile (lower HDL-cholesterol, high triglycerides and usually elevated total cholesterol). In addition abdominal obesity and hypertension are often present. Persons with metabolic syndrome have a marked risk of developing overt diabetes, heart disease, atherosclerosis and stroke.   Metabolic syndrome is in epidemic proportions in all populations that are wealthy enough to eat a modern calorific diet while maintaining relatively sedentary work and life styles. Europeans have decided to find a solution with the LIPGENE research project [208, 209]. The goal is to develop a strategy to alter dietary patterns to prevent metabolic syndrome. European estimates suggest that 10-20% of current middle-aged and elderly men and 10-25% of middle-aged to elderly women have metabolic syndrome. US statistics are much higher, perhaps twice this rate.

Table 5.1. Symptoms of the Metabolic Syndrome (3 or more)

Waistline in women	> 35 inches
-in men	> 40 inches
Blood pressure	> 135/85 mm Hg
Fasting blood glucose	> 110 mg/dl
HDL cholesterol-women	< 50 mg/dl
-men	< 40 mg/dl
Fasting triglycerides	> 150 mg/dl

The higher rates in the USA may have developed because our economy was not as affected by WWII, and we invented and embraced "fast food" before the Europeans. The movie "Super Size Me" depicts a man who put himself into severe metabolic syndrome in just 30 days by eating a fast food diet. One point illustrated particularly well in "Super Size Me" is that *it is easier to get into metabolic syndrome than to get out again.* If we eat our way into metabolic syndrome, is it possible to eat our way out? The answer is partly yes, but the longer the lard stays on, the harder it gets to reverse all damage that has been done.

Reversing Metabolic Syndrome Dr. Gerald Reaven suggests a diet that is 15% protein, 45% carbohydrate, 20% monounsaturated fat, 10% polyunsaturated fat, and less than 10% saturated fat for postmenopausal women [207]. Losing weight by both exercise and caloric control are required for success. It is very helpful to include whole grains, fruits, berries and vegetables in this diet plan so that protective phytochemicals are taken in each day.

Can dietary selections within the recommended macronutrients make a big difference in reversing metabolic syndrome? We believe the answer is YES. Metabolic syndrome is one tough *hombre* and it needs a dedicated diet plan that is packed with phytochemicals and not calories. Food supplements and nutraceuticals have an advantage in highly fortifying the diet without contributing more calories. Evidence to date suggests that phytochemicals can be beneficial in all these ways:

1. **Enhancing insulin action**
2. **Decreasing blood glucose**
3. **Decreasing insulin resistance**
4. **Protecting large blood vessels**
5. **Protecting capillary integrity**
6. **Decreasing formation of AGE proteins**

7. **Decreasing oxidative stress**

8. **Having anti-inflammatory actions**

9. **Decreasing the oxidizability and oxidation of LDL-cholesterol**

10. **Relaxing blood vessels and lowering blood pressure**

Diabetes/Obesity Epidemic Among Native Americans on Modern Diets- What is happening to our entire population was first seen in smaller subgroups of people who converted from active lives with traditional whole foods to sedentary lives with calorific, highly refined, high carbohydrate and high fat diets. Diabetes was unknown in Native Americans until they converted to diets high in refined fats, sugars and starches. The epidemic started around 1900 in some tribes and was in full swing by 1950. Most Native American tribes were confined to reservations where they could not live by the old ways, which included eating wild food and having to work to get it. They once ate Indian corn that they roasted or dried and ground to make flour. Their diet included beans and squash that they raised themselves instead of lard, vegetable oils, white flour and cheese provided by a government surplus program. American Indians ate wild fish and lean venison and wild ducks and turkeys and bear and buffalo. The old-timers harvested wild berries, grapes and nuts, acorns, Indian potatoes and all kinds of green plants and herbals. They would make soup from yellow-jacket grubs or grasshopper cakes mixed with buffalo fat and berries. And they were accustomed to going without food during part of the winter, even surviving on tree bark in tough times. They may not have eaten fewer calories, but they worked hard. It was not uncommon for them to need 3000-4000 Calories a day just to stay even. A simpler, active and more traditional way of life is known to prevent metabolic syndrome. This is a lesson we all need to relearn.

Muscadine phytochemicals and blood glucose control- Remember that the major phytochemicals in muscadines and other grapes are concentrated in the grape skins and grape seeds. There are already several hundred publications in the medical literature describing beneficial effects of these chemicals on blood glucose control and on other effects of diabetes, for example [210-229]. Clifford [230] reviewed the literature on dietary phenols, polyphenols and tannins of the kind found in muscadine grapes. He concluded that one of the most promising benefits of these compounds would be in improving blood glucose control and treating symptoms of the Metabolic Syndrome. Flavonols and polyphenols in grape seeds and skins slow sugar absorption, increase the activity of insulin, and tend to reduce blood sugar [215, 218, 222, 226].

Recently, muscadine juice and muscadine wine were shown to have a positive effect in Type II diabetes. Banini et al. reported at the 2004 Experimental Biology Meeting that individuals were asked to drink either 150 ml of muscadine juice or muscadine wine for 4 weeks. Both healthy and Type II

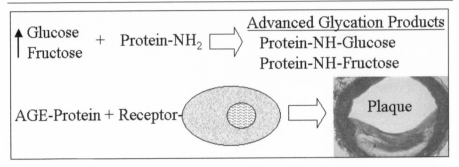

Figure 5.1. Elevated glucose and fructose react with proteins to form Advanced Glycation End-Products that damage blood vessels and other organs.

diabetic subjects were studied. They found that diabetic subjects consuming muscadine wine had a greater decrease in fibrinogen than the diabetics drinking muscadine juice [217]. Fibrinogen is a protein involved in blood clotting. Lowering its levels is considered to be a beneficial effect in cardiovascular risk profiles. Both muscadine juice and muscadine wine decreased blood glucose levels in the diabetic subjects. The effect was greater with muscadine wine than muscadine juice [217]. These results have not appeared in full publication yet, so ref [217] will help you search for these authors in the future.

Muscadines Are Powerful Choices For Metabolic Syndrome- Grape seed extract and related phytochemicals have the potential to help with weight control [231-233]. Maintaining a healthy weight is the single most important step in treating Type II diabetes. Phytochemicals of the kind found in muscadines can improve cholesterol status in the blood and help slow aging of the cardiovascular system [202, 234]. They are also thought to block glycation of proteins and formation of AGE products [235, 236] (Figure 5.1). Procyanidins protect the heart and lower triglycerides [156, 237-239], and high triglycerides is one of the symptoms of the metabolic syndrome. The phytochemicals help prevent blood clotting, which can potentially reduce the incidence of heart attacks and strokes [158, 240, 241]. Grape phytochemicals also protect nerve cells against damage [242], and nerve damage is one of the major problems in diabetes.

Diabetes also causes increased production of free radicals, so the antioxidant effects of muscadine phytochemicals help protect the tissues against this kind of damage [210, 222]. Muscadine grape seed chemicals can block the action of an enzyme that produces part of the damage, especially in the lens of the eye. [243, 244]. One theory suggests that these phytochemicals can help prevent cataracts [228].

The Polyol Pathway Damages Organs- There is strong evidence from animal studies that aldose reductase, the rate-limiting and first enzyme in the polyol pathway plays a key role in damaging small blood vessels in diabetes. The polyol pathway is highly activated under conditions of high blood glucose.

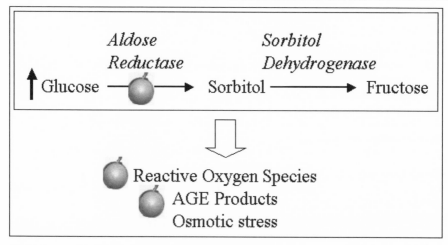

Figure 5.2. In diabetes, glucose is elevated. This activates the polyol pathwy of sorbitol synthesis, which leads to tissue injury. Muscadine phytochemicals counteract this effect by inhibiting aldose reductase and interfering with the formation of AGE products.

It converts excessive glucose to fructose via a sorbitol intermediate. Glucose and fructose both combine with $-NH_2$ groups on proteins (e.g., lysine residues) to form fructosamines (Figure 5.1). One result is an accelerated rate of forming AGE proteins (AGE = Advanced Glycation Endproducts). Glycation means attaching a sugar unit to another large molecule, like proteins. AGE proteins are formed in the walls of all blood vessels and in every organ. This accelerates the aging of every blood vessel and every organ. Most long-term diabetics develop microvascular diseases such as retinopathy, nephropathy and neuropathy. AGE proteins are part of diabetic kidney disease, diabetic atherosclerosis, diabetic peripheral vascular disease, diabetic neuropathies and are highly involves in diabetic cataract formation and retinopathies. Cataracts are opacities that form in the lens of the eye and prevent light from properly reaching the retina. The lens of the eye is particularly sensitive to diabetic damage because it has more aldose reductase than any other organ in the body. It is a marker system for damage that is occurring more silently in all other organs of the body.

Muscadine Phytochemicals Alleviate Complications of Diabetes- A diagram of the Polyol Pathway is shown in Fig. 5.2. Notice that the first enzyme that converts glucose to sorbitol is called aldose reductase. Its level is highly increased under conditions of high blood glucose. It is an advantage to block this enzyme in order to keep glucose from entering this pathway.

Muscadines contain several phytochemicals that are good aldose reductase inhibitors. Ellagic acid has been shown to be one of the most potent inhibitors of aldose reductase in the test tube and in animal studies [224, 245-250]. Ellagic acid at a dose of 75 mg/kg/d inhibited sorbitol accumulation in erythrocytes, lens and sciatic nerves at 50, 75 and 100 mg/kg/d in vivo in diabetic rats [246].

Similarly, kaempferol [47], myricetin [251], myricetin glycosides[50,166], quercetin [252], quercetin glycosides[252] chlorogenic acid [50] and epicatechin[50] inhibit aldose reductase. All are found in muscadines. In addition to direct inhibition of aldose reductase, many muscadine phenolics can inhibit the activation of NF-kappa B and protein kinase C, both known to be involved in gene expression of aldose reductase[253].

A daily serving of foods with these phenolics is important to anyone trying to control blood glucose. This includes anyone considered diabetic, prediabetic, obese or exhibiting metabolic syndrome. If one has been prescribed drugs for any of these conditions, it is important to work with the health professional to insure that proper integrative medicine is achieved. The goal of most highly coordinated programs is to work holistically with the patient to achieve a reversal of the disease state as far as possible and to reduce the drug burden. Reversal is achieved by diet, exercise, stress reduction and integrative medical care. We would argue that drug burden can be reduced most effectively by achieving superior nutrition and well-advised nutraceutical support by a trained professional.

More Anti-Diabetic Effects of Muscadine Phytochemicals- Other activities of muscadine phytochemicals that help manage metabolic syndrome are to reduce blood glucose, increase insulin sensitivity, improve blood lipids, decrease hemoglobin glycosylation, combat oxidative stress and decrease enzymes involved in inflammatory responses. Several of the phytochemicals listed above block the inflammatory enzymes called COX II and 5-LOX. In addition, muscadine skins are extremely high in pectin. It is well known that this soluble fiber can decrease blood glucose by altering the rate of glucose absorbed per unit time after a meal.

Resveratrol and pterostilbene [67, 254], polyphenolic extract of red wine [219], polyphenolic extract of white wine[255], grape seed derived proanthocyanidins [256-258], myricetin [259, 260], chlorogenic acid [261-264], the catechins [265-267], kaempferol [212, 215, 236, 268, 269], OPCs[214] and the anthocyanins [270-275]each has anti-diabetic effects.

Muscadines For People With Diabetes- When people first taste muscadines or try muscadine juice, they often remark about how sweet it tastes. If someone in their family is diabetic, they say, "Oh, it is so good, but my husband (or wife) could never have this, he or she has diabetes." In reality, muscadines and muscadine juice and muscadine wine might actually be allowed in a prediabetic, diabetic or metabolic syndrome diet because of important phytochemicals. One word of caution when buying muscadine juice, **buy 100% muscadine grape juice for diabetic diets**. There are "cider" or beverage products on the market that contain part sugar water and part muscadine juice. Similarly, sugar-added jams, jellies, preserves and other sugar-added products should not be used by diabetics. Muscadine grapes already have Mother Nature's combination of fructose, glucose and some sucrose in just the right amount and in combination with other constituents to make it low glycemic index and low glycemic load. Diabetics and readers battling metabolic syndrome will be familiar with these terms.

Muscadines and the Diabetes Exchange Lists- Diabetes educators have developed a plan called the Exchange System for helping people with diabetes control their blood sugar. A person gets a certain number of food exchanges per day in each food group. In the fruit group, ½ cup of berries (including muscadine grapes) is an exchange. According to a nutritional analysis done by Dr. Betty Ector and posted at the North Carolina Grape Council (see Web Resources), 100 g of muscadines with the seeds removed contains 12-14 g of carbohydrates, 3 g of dietary fiber, no fat and only 68-76 Calories.

1/3 cup of grape juice is an exchange. It is our belief that a person with diabetes might enjoy half a cup of 100% muscadine juice and not have a problem, for at least two reasons. First, the natural sugars are not all converted to glucose in the body. Fructose does not raise blood sugar. Second, the muscadine contains natural fruit acids like malic acid (the same kind that is in apples). Acids slow absorption of sugars. And the phytochemicals also affect glucose usage in the body. If you have diabetes, talk with your diabetes educator or dietitian and ask their opinion for inclusion of muscadines, 100% muscadine juice and muscadine wines into your individualized blood glucose control plan.

Benefit/Risk Ratio is Favorable for Muscadine Products- At present, there is no information suggesting that muscadines or any other whole grape product is a problem for people who are overweight, have diabetes, or any aspect of the metabolic syndrome. The key to Type II diabetes and obesity is balancing portions of foods and beverages and daily activity, plus maintaining a healthy body weight. Muscadines may not be the cure for these conditions, but if used with care, they can be part of the treatment. Meantime, go walking, get your 10,000 steps a day (if foot health permits), and you will be able to refresh yourself with muscadine grape juice. People with Type II diabetes say they can go walking and watch their blood glucose drop back towards the normal range.

Web Resources

American Diabetes Association (Exchange lists and other information for diabetes): http://www.diabetes.org/home.jsp

American Dietetic Association (diet counseling and diabetes education): http://ww.w.eatright.org

North Caroline Grape Council/Muscadine Nutrition: http://www.ncwine.org/muscadine/muscadinenutrition.html

SuperSize Me, www.supersizeme.com

Chapter 6

Muscadines vs. Cancer

The National Cancer Institute educates the public to prevent cancers by making a lifetime commitment to eating a diet enriched with phytochemicals. Prevention is the major line of defense against all cancers. In 1995 a large study in California really prompted coalitions of organizations to come onboard with the chemopreventive message about high fruit and vegetable intake [276]. The National Cancer Institute has really organized and spearheaded research efforts on substances, extracts and combination of ingredient natural products that are chemopreventive. NCI is currently funding a phase II clinical trial to test whether a grape seed extract can improve breast cancer outcomes. There are many phenolics in muscadines that are anti-cancer via one mechnism or combination of mechanisms. In addition, evidence is accumulating that some of these substances can act synergistically within cell signalling systems [277-280]. Because of the number of compounds and the huge literature database, we will limit our review of the literature to those which have been most studied: ellagic acid, quercetin and resveratrol.

How Colon Cancer Develops- The surface of the colon is normally a smooth membrane with tube-shaped glands called crypts that dip under the top layer (Figure 6.1). Cells at the bottom of the crypts divide to replace cells up on the surface that die. It is a harsh place to live and cells live only about a week before being sloughed off. It is the rapidly dividing cells that make us susceptible to cancer, because DNA mutations almost always take place during cell division. The reason is that the DNA has to replicate before the cell divides, and that is an opportunity to get a mutation. If a gene involved in growth or cell division mutates, the daughter cells may not appear normal. The earliest stage of abnormal growth is a microscopic change called the aberrant crypt focus (Figure 6.1). If another mutation occurs, the cells may not slough off, but may divide and pile up on the surface, possibly forming a mushroom-shaped polyp. That is one of the things doctors are looking for when they do colonoscopies. Polyps usually grow slowly, and if they are removed surgically, the source of danger is mostly removed. That is why colonoscopies save lives, because if the polyps are not removed, sometimes another mutation can occur and produce an adenocarcinoma. At this stage, the problem is not a mutation in a single base pair of DNA, because the chromosomes become unstable and can produce mutations by abnormal recombination. Adenomas are still

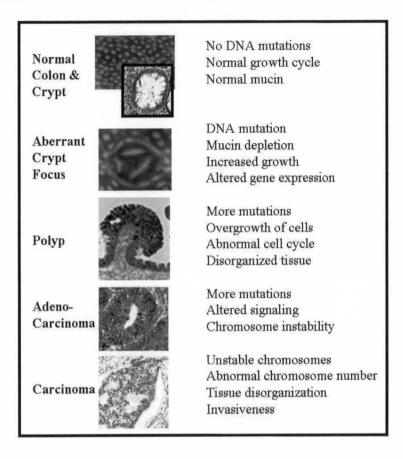

Normal Colon & Crypt		No DNA mutations Normal growth cycle Normal mucin
Aberrant Crypt Focus		DNA mutation Mucin depletion Increased growth Altered gene expression
Polyp		More mutations Overgrowth of cells Abnormal cell cycle Disorganized tissue
Adeno-Carcinoma		More mutations Altered signaling Chromosome instability
Carcinoma		Unstable chromosomes Abnormal chromosome number Tissue disorganization Invasiveness

Figure 6.1. Colon cancers begin when normal cells acquire DNA mutations that cause them to grow more rapidly than needed. As more mutations are acquired, chromosomes become unstable. Colon tissue progresses through at least 5 stages from normal to a microscopic condition called aberrant crypt foci. This may progress to a growth called a polyp that is usually benign, but it may become a dangerous adenocarcinoma. When this breaks through tissue barriers, it can become a carcinoma that spreads to other parts of the body.

attached to the wall of the colon, but if they mutate and become an adenocarcinoma or carcinoma, they can break through the wall of the colon and get in the blood stream or lymph channels. Then they can move up to the liver or into bone and wreak havoc. The progression is similar in other cancers such as breast cancer and liver cancer, but the genes involved are different. Fortunately, several phytochemicals in muscadines and other berries and crucifers help prevent the beginnings of cancer from taking place.

Ellagic Acid in Chemoprevention of Cancer- Muscadine grapes are a rich source of ellagic acid. Ellagic acid is a dimeric derivative of gallic acid. It exists in muscadines, muscadine wines and muscadine juice [43]. In recent years the biomedical importance of ellagic acid in the diet has largely been emphasized by the profound effects that fruit extracts have in preventing various cancers of the gastrointestinal system. Today, ellagic acid and its derivatives are being aggressively investigated for chemoprevention. "Chemoprevention" is a scientific term meaning to chemically prevent cancer from occurring or growing or metastasizing. **Do not confuse chemoprevention with chemotherapy!** Chemotherapy is the use of powerful drugs in protocols designed to arrest and kill various cancers or at least to shrink them in order to buy more time for the patient. Chemoprevention eliminates the need for chemotherapy because the cancer will not occur and therefore the toxic drugs will never be called upon for chemotherapy. Chemoprevention is the ultimate solution to reduce the incidence and lethality of various cancers. Chemoprevention is also geared toward preventing reoccurence of a cancer, decreasing risk of metastasis and prevention of new cancer types in any individual who battles a cancer. Chemoprevention is complementary. The educational programs ongoing by major health institutes to get Americans eating a diet enriched with fruits and vegetables instead of processed foods is designed to provide chemoprevention. The National Cancer Institute estimates that longterm poor dietary habits support or cause a large proportion of various cancer types. NCI highly promotes a high intake of fruits and vegetables with a wide spectrum of chemopreventive phytochemicals to prevent various types of cancer.

Ellagic Acid vs. Cancers- The profound activity of ellagic acid (and its derivatives) in cancer chemoprevention is highly documented by the work of Dr. Gary D. Stoner and colleagues at Ohio State University. Dr. Stoner's work [281-309] has demonstrated that ellagic acid is chemopreventive, and that extracts of fruits containing ellagic acid derivatives are even more powerful than the individual purified substances. This is because there are multiple phenolic substances in a fruit that can act synergistically with the ellagic acid compounds within the complex biological processes that involve cancer initiation, promotion, growth and metastasis. This provides a powerful rationale for following the recommendation to eat an anti-cancer diet instead of relying upon purified substances as single bullets. Much of Dr. Stoner's early work was on ellagic acid as a chemical, then on naturally occurring forms of ellagic acid and finally on enriched ellagic acid sources from fruit extracts containing a synergistic mixture of phenolic phytochemicals. Dr. Stoner's work involves *in vitro* (in the test tube) anti-cancer screening tests, *in vivo* anti-cancer tests in animal models and most recently, clinical trials in humans. Ellagic acid is abundant in certain berries such as raspberries, black raspberries, strawberries, muscadines (muscadines are berries) and in walnuts. Researchers at the Hollings Cancer Center in the Medial University of South Carolina in

Charleston have shown that high ellagic acid fruit extracts, including muscadine extract, inhibit a proteinase that is active in cancers [310, 311].

Dr. Stoner's work provides evidence that ellagic acid will inhibit the development of certain chemically-induced cancers in multiple model systems[294]. Among these are animal models used commonly in the pharmaceutical industry to screen drug activities. He and his colleagues have tested ellagic acid-containing fruit extracts in the chemoprevention of esophageal cancer, colon cancer, and lung cancer. He has also demonstrated that ellagic acid can inhibit the growth of premalignant and malignant oral cell lines. This means that many buccal cancers that are probably initiated by chemicals in food or tobacco can potentially be prevented by exposing the oral cavity to a rinse of ellagic acid containing fruit extracts. Eating a diet containing chemopreventive substances can treat the oral cavity by interacting directly with the surface cells and indirectly via the blood stream after substances get absorbed into the blood via the small intestine. Thus, muscadine and other fruits can be both topically effective and these effects can act synergistically with the systemic effects of a diet enriched with these phytochemicals. Considering the devastating effects of oral cancer, a bowl of fruit a day seems like a very logical chemoprevention protocol

Ellagic Acid Prevents Mutagenesis or Initiation of Multiple Cancers- In summarizing the effects of ellagic acid in cancer studies, it is important to realize that cancers have different stages of intervention. Briefly, there is the initiation or mutagenesis phase, a promotional phase and a metastatic phase. Ellagic acid prevents mutagenesis, the process that inititiates cancer. There are many known carcinogens (substances that initiate cancers) that are used experimentally. Ellagic acid has been demonstated to reduce both the mutagenicity and carcinogenicity of many of these agents: 4-(methyl-nitrosamino)-1-(3-pyridyl)-1-butanone [208,[312]]; aflatoxin B1 [305]; 3-amino-1-methyl-5Hpyriso[4,3-b]indole [208, 225]; benzo[a]pyrene [313, 314]; 3-methylcholanthrene[315, 316]; N-2-fluorenylacetamide [317, 318]; N-methyl-N-nitrosurea [319]; N-nitrosodimethylamine [319]; 7,12-dimethyl-benz[a]anthracene [320]; N-nitrosobenzylmethylamine[303, 304] and pulmonary carcinogenesis induced by NNK, a carcinogen in cigarettes[321], and methylbenzyl nitrosamine[322]. The above have been demonstrated in skin, tongue, esophageal, mammary, gastric, esophageal, colon and duodenal cancers in rodents [208][323]. In a salmon model for screening pre-initiation and post-initiation anti-cancer effects in multiple organs, ellagic acid suppressed stomach cancer incidence and multiplicity when fed after initiation with a carcinogen called DMBA (7,12-dimethyl-benz[a]anthracene. There was also a growth rate suppression observed in remaining tumors[290]. In a microsome-mediated test system for testing chemoprevention, ellagic acid inhibited the formation of DNA adducts both directly and indirectly [324]. Others have reported that ellagic acid bound to DNA can inhibit the induction of esophageal cancer caused by MBN (methylbenzylnitrosamine)[322, 325]. Ellagic acid in the drinking water decreased the mutagenicity of NMBA (N-nitrosomethylbenzylamine) in a rat model of esophageal cancer [326]. Ellagic acid also inhibits the conversion of ethanol to acetaldehyde in breast tissue. Since ethanol consumption has been linked to a higher incidence of breast cancer, this effect of ellagic acid can be considered a chemopreventive action [327].

Ellagic Acid Induces Detoxification Enzymes Ellagic acid induces gene expression of an enzyme called NAD(P)H:quinone reductase(QR) [312]. This enzyme is involved in the detoxification of carcinogens and thereby an induction of gene expression for this enzyme will decrease the mutagenesis and tumorigenesis of a battery of carcinogens. In rats fed ellagic acid there was a 9-fold increase in hepatic and a 2-fold increase in pulmonary QR activity [225]. Ellagic acid is a powerful antioxidant. An antioxidant responsive element controls the QR gene expression. The same researchers demonstrated that the QR gene expression was induced by ellagic acid [225]. This represents another powerful effect of ellagic acid on gene expression relevant to cancer prevention.

Anti-Proliferative Effects of Ellagic Acid in Cancer Test Systems Ellagic acid has been shown to be anti-proliferative in Caco-2 cells (colon cancer), MCF-7 cells (breast cancer), Hs578T cells (breast cancer) and DU145 cells (prostatic cancer cells)[328]. Of these, Caco-2 colon cancer cells were most sensitive and MCF-7 breast cancer cells were least sensitive [238]. In addition, these investigators showed that ellagic acid impairs the HUVEC (blood vessel endothelial cell) cell tube formation and proliferation [238]. This process is necessary to continually form blood vessels to supply growing tumors. In addition, ellagic acid was shown to produce apoptosis (programmed cell death) in the cancer cell lines without inducing apoptosis in normal cells. Ellagic acid has been shown to arrest the cell cycle, inhibit overall cell growth and induce apoptosis in CaSki cells (cervical cancer) after 72 hours of treatment[311]. Of perhaps greater importance is the probability that ellagic acid acts synergistically with other phytochemicals to augment the anti-cancer effects of each. Such an effect has been demonstrated in MOLT-4 human leukemia cells [279, 280, 282, 329].

Absorption of Ellagic Acid Compounds One thing of concern with any substance is whether it can be absorbed well enough to get to necessary sites of action. For ellagic acid, this is especially true because ellagic acid itself is poorly absorbed through the gut wall[282]. On the other hand, many of the gastrointestinal tract cancers that can be suppressed by ellagic acid, can be treated via the gut side. So ellagic acid can potentially suppress oral cancers, esophageal, stomach, small intestine and colon cancers because it is in the gut and in contact with the lining cells of the gastrointestinal tract. Indeed, Stoner et al have recently demonstrated that these epithelial cells can concentrate ellagic acid [282] Most ellagic acid is in foods in the form of ellagitannins. These are a group of many larger molecules that yield ellagic acid when they are broken down by hydrolysis reactions that can take place in the body. Molecules that appear in the blood and in the urine can be quite different than the molecules ingested in the food because the body has so many ways to metabolize substances and modify their stuctures. A suggested marker for ellagitannins is urolithin B. Researchers recently reported that this metabolite of ellagic acid increases markedly in urine when intake of ellagitannin is increased in the diet of humans[330]. Much of the urolithin B may be made by normal colon bacteria. Therefore, the ellagitannins have probably treated the entire gastrointestinal tract before they get converted to the urolithin B. Urolithin B is also bioactive and can therfore have beneficial effects as it circulates before excretion. Urolithin B has antiangiogenic and hyaluronidase inhibition activities, two very important anti-cancer properties [242, [331]. While a percentage of ellagic acid does get absorbed higher in the GI tract, it appears in the blood as metabolites and not as free ellagic acid [332]. These metabolites may be bioactive as they circulate in the body. Only a small fraction of ellagic acid gets absorbed into the bloodstream in the upper intestine. However, this can be augmented by the metabolites originating in the lower GI tract. In summary, the entire GI tract can benefit from the ingestion of ellagic acid and ellagic acid compounds.

A recent review article summarized the mechanisms by which phenolic phytochemicals can interupt proliferation of cancer cells in known molecular biological pathways[277]. Ellagic acid is one of these compounds known to inhibit the activation of redox-sensitive transcription factors. These transcription factors are NF-kB, AP-1 and c-myc. Ellagic acid may interact with all three of these systems. It is known that ellagic acid inhibits the activation of NF-kB. In addition, these compounds can inhibit the activation of MAPK (mitogen-activated protein kinase). NF-kB activation controls gene expression of COX-2 gene. AP-1 controls gene expression of metalloproteinase genes and c-myc controls expression of cyclin B1 genes. These genes are each involved in the mechanisms the lead to enhanced cell cycle progression needed to sustain cancer cell proliferation and tumor growth [245]. Ingestion of diets rich in these phenolic phytochemicals is a matter of public education by the National Cancer Institute to prevent and decrease the incidence of many cancers.

Resveratrol and Its Family of Compounds in Chemoprevention of Cancer

Resveratrol and its derivatives are chemopreventive in assays representing three major stages of carcinogenesis: tumor initiation, promotion and progression [333, 334]. Resveratrol is also anti-metastatic, antioxidant and antimutagenic.

Some compounds are not carcinogenic until they have been metabolized by enzymes called cytochrome P450s (2). Resveratrol has been shown to inhibit the expression of certain cytochrome P450s, inhibit their activity (20,21) and can also induce detoxification Phase II enzymes. These Phase II enzymes metabolize xenobiotics and thereby transform mutagenic compounds into less toxic substances. One of these Phase II enzymes is call NAD(P)H:quinone reductase. Resveratrol and ellagic acid have each been demonstrated to increase the gene expression and the cellular activity of this enzyme[335, 336].

Resveratrol and Apoptosis Resveratrol also helps regulate the cell cycle. If DNA is damaged, it can either be repaired or cell systems can program the cell to die. If a cell has undergone DNA damage leading to a cancerous mutation, it is obviously desirable for that cell to die. Programmed cell death is called "apoptosis" by scientists. Resveratrol is a substance that helps stop mutated cells from propogating. Resveratrol stimulates these cells toward the "apoptosis" mechanism. This is a very desirable and anti-cancer effect since cancer cells are so effective at propogating. Resveratrol has been shown in several cancer cell types to induce cell cycle arrest, inhibit cancer cell proliferation and actually induce apoptosis See [337] for review of a large body of biomedical literature.

Inhibition of Gene Expression for Metalloproteinases by Inhibition of NF-kappa B Activation In animal model of tumor growth, resveratrol also exhibits acitivities that would tend to diminish tumor growth and tumor metastasis. In order for a tumor to grow, it needs to "create space" for itself to grow. Otherwise, the pressure of normal tissue would limit the tumor severely. Obviously, tumors have ways to occupy space that is normally occupied by normal cells. One mechanism that tumor cells use to create space involves secretion of some enzymes called "metalloproteinases". Again, another unfriendly scientific term. What these enzymes do is to dissolve or degrade the connective matrix around normal cells in the neighborhood. The normal cell will then be "pushed aside" or they will die because their environment is disrupted. Resveratrol has been shown to downregulate gene expression of metalloproteinase [137, 338]. Inhibition of metalloproteinases has been shown using muscadine extracts[335]and wine polyphenols[339]. Piceatannol, a resveratrol analog, has been shown to inhibit both activation of NF-kappa B and gene expression for NF-kappaB[134]. NF-kappa B activation stimulates gene expression for metalloproteinases. In fact, many of the phytochemicals in muscadines are known to inhibit activation of NF-kappaB: Resveratrol[131, 132, 135, 137, 340], procyanidins [341], several of the flavonoids[342-349] the anthocyanins[179, 350, 351]and the phenolic acids[352-355].

Inhibition of Angiogenesis As tumor cells proliferate and the tumor begins to grow, it also needs to ensure that blood vessels grow along with it to keep it supplied with food, oxygen and to carry away waste products. Without this happening, the tumor would rapidly shrink and disappear as all its cells would die. The process of promoting blood vessel growth is called "angiogenesis". It is regulated by a complex set of signals between the tumor cells and the existing blood vessel cells. Resveratrol is an angiogenesis inhibitor [356-366] in various in vitro and in vivo tests for this effect. This is an effect shared by many other phytochemicals in muscadines and grapes in general[358]. Ellagic acid[367]and the flavonoids[368, 369] also have anti-angiogenic activity.

Other evidence of the anti-cancer activities of the phytochemicals found in muscadines comes from cancer cell culture screens and an impressive number of animal models of tumorigenesis, tumor promotion and tumor metastasis.

Quercetin and the Flavonols Quercetin is a flavanol that is found in muscadine grapes and in onions, apples, red wine, black tea, buckwheat tea, and Ginkgo biloba. Like resveratrol, quercetin is an excellent antioxidant and is anti-inflammatory. It protects against DNA mutations, colon cancer and heart disease [370]. In humans, protection against carcinogenesis is the best documented effect of flavonols [371]. Quercetin and two relatives called kaempferol and myricetin are concentrated in muscadine skins at about 1.1-6.8 mg/100 g fresh weight [43, 192]. Because the daily intake of all flavanols is about 20-23 mg [370, 372], muscadine nutraceutical products can be a significant source of these compounds.

In natural, whole foods quercetin is mostly attached to glucose or other sugars. Whereas quercetin itself is poorly absorbed, quercetin glucosides are taken up into the body by means of a sugar transporter [373, 374]. They are conjugated in the body to produce a glucuronide, so that neither quercetin nor quercetin glucoside is present at significant concentrations in blood. Several other compounds are produced from flavanols in the intestinal tract [375], and it is not clear which of these compounds is responsible for protective effects. Some of the metabolites have actions that are similar to quercetin itself but are milder [376]. The highest amount of flavonols found in the blood after eating foods or pure quercetin glucosides is about 1-7 μM, and the compounds persist for several days because their half lives are about 10-28 hours [371, 377]. Grapes contain mixtures of quercetin glucosides and other glycosides [193], but the relative amounts of these compounds in muscadines has not been published.

Muscadines versus cancer- Whole muscadines are unusual among grapes because they contain significant amounts of ellagic acid and quercetin. The only other common fruits and berries that have this combination are strawberries, raspberries and blackberries. Although blueberries have both chemicals, the amount of ellagic acid is small [278]. The reason this combination is significant is that both phytochemicals combat abnormal cell growth and cancer, but their effects are stronger when they are combined [278-280, 329, 378, 379]. In a line of human leukemia cells, ellagic acid combined with quercetin at levels similar to those found in muscadine wine slowed cell growth and the cell division cycle, and caused the cancer cells to die [379].

Synergism Between Quercetin and Ellagic Acid Recent work has shown that ellagic acid combined with quercetin act together to affect cell controls over the growth rate and the path by which cancer cells die. The combination changes the activity of regulatory proteins and enzymes called MAP kinases that regulate cell division and viability [279, 280].

Catechins and Cancer Prevention Although there is much evidence that tea catechins help prevent several kinds of cancer, it is not clear that the main forms found in muscadines are as effective. Green tea contains a compound called EGCG (epigallocatechin gallate), whereas muscadine seeds contain catechin and epicatechin. However, several other flavonoids in muscadines do have anti-cancer activity in a chemically induced model of breast cancer.

Stilbenes and Cancer Prevention The anti-cancer bioactivities of resveratrol were discussed above. This may be just the beginning for stilbene research in this area. In Figure 3.5 in Chapter 3, the family of resveratrol analogs is shown. Although the names of the compounds make them sound unrelated, a quick look at the chemical structures reveals that they are very closely related. Many of these analogs are made in plants that produce resveratrol. Resveratrol is not necessarily the endgame molecule for plants or humans. When humans ingest these compounds, our own metabolic pathways act on them to convert them to other compounds. For example, resveratrol can be converted to piceatannol in the grape. When absorbed by humans, resveratrol can be converted to piceatannol in the liver by a hydroxylation enzyme. Piceatannol is a very bioactive metabolite[380-384]. E.g., it inhibits the cell cycle of colorectal cancer cells[385]. Similarly, scirpusin, astringin, pterostilbene, the viniferins, resveratroloside and the piceids are bioactive molecules [386]. Scirpusin has significant anti-HIV activity[387]. Astringin has antioxidant and antimutagenic activity[386, 388, 389] and can be increased in grapes with postharvest irradiation with UV light. This is true of some of the other analogs of resveratrol as well. Pterostilbene has several anti-cancer activities[390-393]. The viniferins have anti-inflammatory and anti-cancer activities[394-402]. Reveratroloside has activities that are anti-cancer [386, 403] and it likely human metabolism rapidly removes the glucose unit and reverts this compound back to resveratrol during intestinal absorption. The piceids are also a glucoside of resveratrol and appear in very high concentrations in grapes, grape juices and wines[63, 64, 404-406]. While not studied as well as resveratrol, removal of the glucose unit by glucosidase activity yields free resveratrol and therefore probably shares actions with resveratrol. Piceid has been found to inhibit tumor growth and lung metastasis in Lewis lung carcinoma-bearing mice [407].

Anthocyanins and Proanthocyanidins and Cancer Prevention For example, synergistic or additive antiproliferative actions were found for the anthocyanins, proanthocyanidins, and flavonol glycosides within cranberry extract [408]. A procyanidin fraction from grape seed also shows anti-cancer activity [409]. Increasing numbers of papers are showing that extracts of berries and fruits have more anti-cancer activity than any isolated molecule on its own.

The anthocyanins are the colored pigments that give purple, blue and red berries and flowers their colors. These pigments are formed by addition of a sugar to an anthocyanidins. Juices, wines or the skins of purple muscadines are excellent sources of these compounds (as are other purple and black grapes). In addition, the anthocyanidins combine to form condensed tannins (proanthocyanidins) that are made of 2 or more anthocyanidins combined. Grape seeds are a rich source of OPCs. There are more than 80 publications that discuss the ability of different anthocyanins to prevent different kinds of cancer, and more than 20 references to proanthocyanidins and cancer. For example, consumption of purple grape juice significantly blocked the ability of a chemical carcinogen to damage mammary DNA, and the growth of breast tumors was reduced [410]. Anthocyanidins of the same types found in muscadines have been shown to slow the growth of human stomach, colon, breast, lung and brain cancer cells in a laboratory test [411]. Tests in cell culture and animal models have shown that berry extracts reduce cancer cell growth (or cause increased cancer cell death) in colon cancer, breast cancer, prostate cancer and leukemia models.

Anthocyanidins and proanthocyanidins block cancer development in several ways. For example, the polyphenolics in whole grape juice inhibit DNA synthesis in breast cancer cells [412]. Tumors require growth of new blood vessels to supply their high metabolic activity, but anthocyanidins block blood vessel growth into some tumors [176, 413]. Grape seed extract also blocks drug metabolizing enzymes that may activate carcinogens, and affects the response of cells to tumor necrosis factor-alpha [24] and certain growth factors [414]. Grape seed extract shows promise in helping rescue normal tissues during cancer chemotherapy [415]. It also reduces growth rates of prostate cancer cells [416, 417]. Finally, water extracts of muscadine grapes inhibit the activity of metalloproteinases, enzymes involved in cancer metastasis[310]

Because muscadines are excellent sources of anti-cancer compounds including ellagic acid compounds, resveratrol and its analogs, quercetin and other flavonoids, anthocyanins and proanthocyanidins, muscadine products would make a powerful choice in a cancer prevention diet.

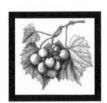

Chapter 7 -

Muscadine Grapes, Inflammation and Arthritis

Inflammation is a Key Process in Multiple Chronic Diseases That Shorten Life- Let us start with good news about preventing many chronic diseases or helping to reverse them. Muscadine grapes and the phytochemicals in juices, wines, pomace, dried muscadine powder, and muscadine seeds or extracts help the body repair itself. They are good for your heart and blood vessels, good for the internal organs as well as the digestive system, good for joints, immune system, brain and connective tissue. Aging may be graceful or accelerated and ungraceful. Aging slowly is desirable in order to attain greater longevity with higher quality of life in senior years. Accelerated aging occurs in chronic disease states that involve systemic inflammation.

System-wide inflammation may be present in high oxidative stress states, heart disease, blood vessel disease, diabetes, obesity, metabolic syndrome and cancers. Inflammation is natural and desirable up to a point when there is injury to tissues, invasion by bacteria or foreign substancex. Once a local inflammation goes systemic, it first involves blood vessels and then the cells of organs such as the heart, kidneys, and eyes. Cells of the immune system are the major players in inflammation. It is important to support healthy immune system function, but to prevent the immune system from over responding and triggering a vicious cycle that grows out of control. Many inflammatory conditions will have the suffix "itis" attached to their names, e.g., arthritis, gingivitis, prostatitis, mastitis, dermatitis, vasculitis, neuritis, bronchitis, enteritis, colitis, hepatitis, pancreatitis. When you get a bad case of any of these conditions, they can make the your whole body feel miserable because toxic substances and signals like cytokines get released into the blood stream and lead to aches and pains at sites distant from the original inflammation (Figure 7.1).

Abdominal Fat Makes Inflammation Worse- Inflammation is a condition caused by cells of the immune system and the tissues with which they interact. Fat cells are part of this system and release many products that make inflammation and many diseases worse. For example, immune cells communicate by sending out protein messengers called cytokines. Literally, the word cytokine means "to stimulate a cell." Fat cells in the abdominal cavity produce the cytokines called tumor necrosis factor α and interleukins 6 and 8, which are classic cytokines that are also made by cells of the immune system.

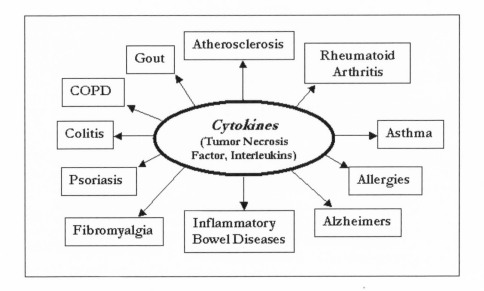

Figure 7.1. Anti-inflammatory actions of phytochemicals in muscadines suppress cytokine release. Cytokines are major players in multiple chronic inflammatory diseases.

Fat cells also produce several proteins that contribute to elevated blood cholesterol, such as cholesterol ester transfer protein or CETP (Figure 7.2). Angiotensinogen II is a precursor of a hormone that elevates blood pressure called angiotensin II. Fat cells secrete angiotensinogen in metabolic syndrome[418]. When fat accumulates, sensitivity to insulin declines and blood glucose begins to rise. If fatty acids are too elevated, they can be toxic to some cells. Remember the watchword to keep your waistline under 35 inches if you are a woman and under 40 inches if you are a man. Diet and exercise are the best tools in the fight against metabolic syndrome. Planned activity and sound food choices help keep blood pressure down, lower cholesterol, and reduce the degree of inflammation your system faces. The good news is that one doesn't have to lose all the weight to see significant improvements. Just getting on an appropriate diet and beginning to lose weight with diet and exercise causes marked beneficial metabolic profile changes[419, 420]. See Chapter 5 for more information concerning metabolic syndrome and diabetes.

A Clinical Marker for Systemic Inflammation- C-reactive protein (CRP) is a marker of chronic inflammation that is now measured in blood tests to determine risk for cardiovascular disease. Any time there is a chronic systemic inflammation, the endothelial cell function is impaired and the atherosclerotic process accelerates. That is why most people with chronic inflammatory disease end up dying of heart attacks and strokes. Did you know that CRP

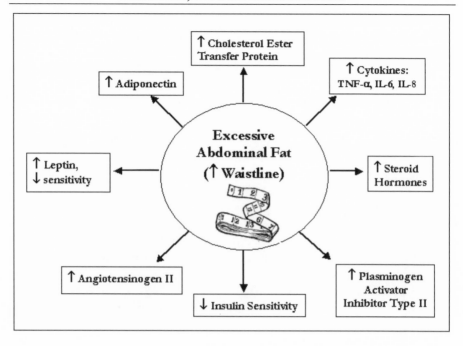

Fig. 7.2. Fat cells in the abdomen produce inflammatory cytokines including tumor necrosis factor-α and interleukins. They also make hormones and enzymes that reduce sensitivity to insulin, raise blood glucose and fatty acids, increase cholesterol and tend to make blood clot. These pathologies constitute metabolic syndrome and can be combated with a tape measure, exercise program and diet plan..

is a much better predictor for who will have a heart attack than is LDL-cholesterol? For an update discussion see[421]. Yes, many people who don't have elevated cholesterols get heart attacks. Their problem is systemic inflammation. The atherosclerotic process can aggressively accumulate LDL into plaque even when it is normal or low in the blood. That is how powerful even low grade systemic inflammation can be in blood vessel health. Other markers for systemic inflammation include fibrinogen levels, homocysteine levels and serum amyloid A levels. If your doctor is ordering these tests, it is a good sign your doctor understands how important these markers are in determining overall health risks. These markers are non-specific, meaning they will go up no matter what kind of infection you have or where it is presently located. A PubMed search on C-reactive protein yielded 71,528 hits.

CRP for Risk Assessment- CRP is thought to be a useful marker in risk stratification for heart attacks and strokes[422, 423]. Out of thousands of articles, we have selected just a few that update the use of these markers in cardiology. These markers are signals in atherosclerotic inflammatory disease. Two reasons that aspirin is recommended for people with atherosclerotic disease is that it is anti-inflammatory and anti-platelet. The trick with atherosclerotic disease is to cool down the inflammation in order to keep plaques from destabilizing and then to keep blood clots from forming. It takes a long time to build a plaque and it may take an even longer time to regress a plaque. The more immediate and practical approach is to stabilize the situation to prevent progression, then work on regression. It is an exciting area of research and it allows a doctor and patient to assess the degree of risk for a given individual much better than traditional risk factors. We suggest the following articles for those who want to understand this better [424-429].

What is Inflammation? By the age of 5, we have all experienced inflammation. When the bee stung you, that was inflammation. If a dog bit you, that was inflammation. If you got cut with a knife or broken glass, ditto. No matter what happened, it caused pain, swelling, redness, warmth in the tissues, and loss of function. Those are the 5 symptoms of inflammation. After a while, the cuts healed over, the pain and swelling went away, and you went on to your next adventure. In other words, the tissues healed themselves. Specifically, immune cells cleaned up the bacteria and foreign matter, the fiber forming cells stitched the tissues together, and the skin grew back over the injured area. A scar might have remained, but you felt as good as new. Defending you and healing you are what the connective tissues are supposed to do. Phytochemicals in muscadine are good choices for an anti-inflammatory diet because the decrease the strength of the inflammation.

Even when you have not had a sting or an injury, these cells are moving around your body, cleaning things up and making repairs. They take care of problems that are so small, you never notice. Who can feel immune cells cleaning up cholesterol? No one can, but it happens. Who can tell when an immune cell has detected a cancer cell and removed it from your system so it will not grow into a large mass? No one, but it happens ever day. So it is important to help out the cells that are trying to help you by eating right, staying active, and not smoking.

Muscadine Anti-inflammatory Power- When you get arthritis and your joints hurt, that is inflammation. There is good news about fighting inflammation. The phytochemicals in muscadines are not just antioxidants, they are also anti-inflammatory. In the first experiment we did with muscadines, an extract of grape skin was compared with a powerful pain reliever for ability to prevent bad cholesterol from becoming oxidized. The muscadine extract was more powerful than the medication! That got our attention.

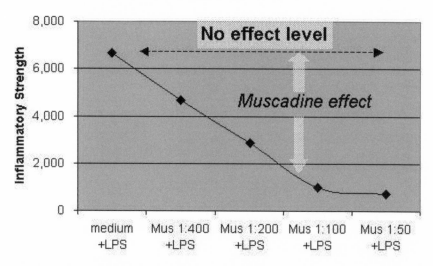

Figure 7.3. Muscadine extract prevents an inflammatory response to a bacterial product called lipopolysaccharide (LPS). In cells treated with LPS alone, the strength of inflammation was more than 6000 units (left side of figure). As dilutions of muscadine extract were added, the response was blocked until at a 1:100 dilution, LPS did not produce this inflammatory response (right side of figure).

Test after test has shown similar results. Figure 7.3 shows one of the typical anti-inflammatory tests using muscadine skin extracts. Human monocytes were grown in a laboratory and treated with an inflammatory drug called LPS. Then the cells released a powerful inflammatory chemical (over 6000 units of PGE2 as shown for "Medium plus LPS'). PGE2 stands for prostaglandin E2. It is a major mediator of inflammatory responses. The arrow labled <u>No Effect Level</u> Indicates what would be expected if there was no response to the muscadine extracts, i.e., all the results would be the same. However, when muscadine extract was added to the cell cultures, much less of the inflammatory chemical was released. Muscadine skin extract was diluted way down for these tests. The Mus 1:400 label means that there were 400 parts solvent to 1 part muscadine skins. The Mus 1:50 is more concentrated at 1 part muscadine skins and 50 parts solvent. What these data indicate is that muscadine skins have very high anti-inflammatory activity. See [430] for full discussion of this experiment.

As shown in Figs. 7.3 and 7.4, the more muscadine extract that is added, the less inflammatory compounds is released from the immune cell. This is called a "dose-response" in medical research. When a bigger response is produced with more muscadine extract (a lesser dilution), it increases the confidence that the results are true. In other words, the muscadine extract produced a dose-dependent response on the secretion of PGE2 from human monocytes. The result indicates that muscadine phytochemicals can lessen the inflammatory response. We emphasize that this was much more dilute than the phytochemicals in whole muscadines, muscadine juice, wine or food

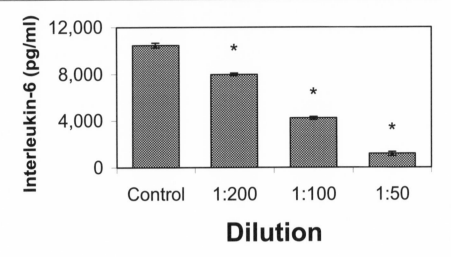

Fig. 7.4. Muscadine extracts decrease the release of cytokines such as interleukin 6 from cultured human monocytes. Asterisks indicate that the change is statistically significant compared to the control value. Data are from Greenspan et al. (2005) with permission.

supplements. While the seeds were not tested in this particular experiment, there is an enormous literature concerning the anti-inflammatory powers of grape seeds and their extracts. Food supplement and nutraceutical products made from the muscadine seeds are highly anti-oxidant and highly anti-inflammatory. Lessening a powerful inflammatory response like that evoked by LPS in the above experiment is a very beneficial effect relevant to human inflammatory diseases.

Effect of Muscadine Extracts on the Release of Cytokines and Superoxide Free Radicals-Researchers at the University of Georgia evaluated the anti-inflammatory activity of muscadine skins in two more anti-inflammation tests. The skins were dried, pulverized and extracted with 50% ethanol [430]. These extracts were tested in two different assays; (1) the production of superoxide free radicals in activated neutrophils, and (2) the release of cytokines by activated human mononuclear cells. The release of superoxide and cytokines by these cell types is part of the inflammatory process.

Effect of Muscadine Extracts on Release of Oxidative Free Radicals by Human Neutrophils- Human neutrophils were incubated with dilutions of muscadine skin extract for 1 hr. The cells were then activated and incubated for another hour and the production of superoxide free radicals was measured. As illustrated in Figure 7.4, a concentration- dependent inhibition of superoxide production was observed. This is a dose-response relationship. A 1:25 final dilution of the muscadine skin extract produced a 94% inhibition in the release of superoxide radicals, while a 1:100 dilution of the extract resulted in an approximately 65% inhibition. For comparison, aspirin (not shown here, but run for comparison purposes) at a concentration of 100 µg/ml, inhibited superoxide production by approximately 70%[430].

Effect of Muscadine Extracts on Release of Cytokines by Human Monocytes- In experiments similar to Figure 7.4, the effect of muscadine skin extracts on the release of two other cytokines, IL-1 and TNF-alpha was studied in activated human peripheral blood mononuclear cells. 24 hours after activation, the cell culture supernatants were assayed for content of IL-1 and TNF-alpha. Again, muscadine skin extracts produced concentration-dependent inhibition in the release of the cytokines. A 1:200 dilution of the muscadine skin extract inhibited the release of TNF-alpha by approximately 15% while a 1:50 dilution produced nearly 90% reduction. The muscadine skin extract was even more potent in its effect on IL-1 release. A 1:400 dilution inhibited IL-1 release by approximately 50% and a 1:200 dilution inhibited the release of IL-1 by 93%. These data further validate muscadine anti-inflammatory power.

Muscadines Suppress Carrageenan-induced Paw Edema- One of the symptoms of inflammation is swelling (edema). The idea that muscadines in the diet would suppress edema was tested by an experiment using rats. Male rats were fed whole muscadine skin powder as 5% of their diet for two weeks. On day 15, the rats were injected with 0.5 mg of carrageenan to cause edema (swelling) in a hind paw. Hind paw volumes (edema) were recorded 3 hr later. Indomethacin and other non-steroidal anti-inflammatory drugs have been shown to suppress carrageenan-induced edema. Rats with muscadine skin powder in the diet had ~50% less paw edema than controls. These results demonstrate that dietary supplementation with whole powdered muscadine skins has marked anti-inflammatory activity *in vivo*.

Many phytochemicals in muscadines are anti-inflammatory and can help lessen the severity of an inflammatory response. Chronic systemic inflammatory responses are very destructive to the body. Lessening systemic inflammation is beneficial in multiple disease states. There are several ways that these phytochemicals can fight inflammation.

Inhibition Of Pro-Inflammatory Signaling By Inhibiting COX II And LOX- Cyclooxygenase II (COXII) is an enzyme that synthesizes prostaglandins from arachidonic acid. Prostaglandins are potent mediators of events involved in inflammation. Gene expression of COX II enzymes is highly increased during inflammatory diseases. Lipoxygenase or LOX is a family of enzymes that convert arachidonic acid to leukotriences that are involved in many inflammatory diseases. Asthma is a primary example. Phytochemicals in muscadines with either anti-COX II or anti-LOX activity or both include: caffeic acid and its derivatives, kaempferol, myricetin, OPCs (oligomeric proanthocyanidins), gallocatechin, epicatechin, piceid, quercetin, resveratrol, and viniferin.

Antioxidant activity scavenges and neutralizes oxidative free radicals-
The phenolic and polyphenolic substances in each fraction of muscadines are antioxidants. Among the prevalent muscadine phenolics with high antioxidant activity are: caffeic acid and its derivatives, chlorogenic acid, catechin, ellagic acid and its derivatives, OPCs (oligomeric proanthocyanidins), piceatannol, epicatechin and its derivatives, the flavonoids in general, gallic acid, kaempferol and its derivatives, quercetin, resveratrol, and the polyphenols in general.

Inhibition of Platelet Activating Factor- Biologically active lipids have been found in wine, juice and wine must (must is unfermented juice, pulp and skins of grapes). Both white and red grapes contain a large number of polar phospho- and glycolipids that can inhibit platelet-activating factor (PAF)[431-434]. This thins the blood and helps prevent blood clotting. Grape seeds are also known to have factors that inhibit platelet aggregation. One report indicated that this effect was comparable to aspirin and was probably due to the procyanidins in the seeds[435]. Muscadine grape seeds are extremely high in OPCs. Inhibition of platelet hyperreactivity is very beneficial for preventing heart attacks and strokes.

Muscadine Phytochemicals Block NF-KB Activation That Controls Scores Of Other Gene Products- Muscadines contain many substances that can block the activation of nuclear factor kappa B (NF-kB) and thereby suppress gene expression for many inflammatory molecules or enzymes. Inhibition of NF-kB activation has been shown for caffeic acid, quercetin, resveratrol and its derivatives, ellagic acid and its derivatives and proanthocyanidins. Inducible nitric oxide synthase (iNOS) gene expression is inhibited by caffeic acid, chlorogenic acid, quercetin, resveratols, proanthocyanidins, OPCs, kaempferol, polyphenols in general, tannic acid, gallotannin. Inducible NOS has also been shown to be inhibitable by myricetin.

Inhibition of leukocyte adhesion and movement mechanisms- When an infection or injury occurs that initiates the inflammatory responses, mechanisms are invoked to signal leukocytes (white blood cells) in the blood to pass out of the blood and into the tissue site where their actions are needed. Monocytes, macrophages and neutrophils are examples of some white blood cells. Anti-inflammation tests were performed on these cell types above. These are cell types that have to move from the blood to the tissue site of inflammation by moving across the lining of the blood vessel. The blood vessel lining is composed of vascular endothelial cells. How do these cells know where to stop and cross the blood vessel lining? How do they actually crawl through the lining? What happens is that signals from the infectious bacteria or products released in response to injury affect gene expression in the vascular endothelial cell. See Figure 4.2 for the general process.

Activated Endothelial Cells Express Cell Adhesion Molecules for Leukocytes- Activated vascular endothelial cells become sticky when they insert more cell adhesion molecules on the blood surface. These are binding proteins called selectins. White blood cells like neutrophils, monocytes and macrophages have receptors (integrins) on their cell surfaces that can interact or bind with the selectins on the endothelial cell surface. White blood cells are ordinary moving very fast with the stream of blood. Interactions between the integrins on the white blood cells and the selectin binding proteins on the walls of the vessel will slow them down to a crawl and then a stop. In this manner, the endothelial cells communicate to the white blood cells that this is the right place to migrate into the tissue. See Figure 4.2. ICAM is one of the cell adhesion molecules on the surface of the activated endothelial cell. ICAM means intercellular adhesion molecule. These interactions form stronger attachments. Using even more attachments between integrins and VCAM-1 and PECAM-1, the white cells are tethered in place and can now pass between the endothelial cells lining the blood vessel. This process is called **"transmigration"**. Monocytes, lymphocytes and all leukocytes use such mechanisms. It is like having sequential velcro attachments that allow the leukocytes to get out of the blood and into the specific site in the tissue. The process is highly controlled by activation of the vascular endothelial cells. See Figure 4.2.

NF-kappa B Activation, Endothelial Cell Activation and Leukocyte Transmigration- Activation of NF-kappa B is highly involved in the processes activating vascular endothelial cells during inflammation. NF-kappa B activation controls gene expression for cell adhesion molecules. Therefore, it is not surprising that most of the substances listed above as inhibitors of NF-kappa B activation will suppress gene expression of cell adhesion molecules by the vascular endothelial cell. In this manner, inhibitors of NF-kappa B activation can suppress transmigration of leukocytes from blood to tissue. Since this basic mechanism is involved in all inflammatory diseases and metastatic cancer, it should be no surprise that these phytochemicals are good preventive medicine for multiple conditions.

Muscadine Phytochemicals Affect Key Players in Inflammation- Suffice it to say that muscadines are a source of many phytochemicals that can suppress activation of the vascular endothelial cell in response to several tested stimuli, reduce gene expression for both cell adhesion molecules and decrease the number of cytokine signaling molecules that are being released. Muscadine protect the health of vascular endothelial cells and decrease the oxidation of harmful LDL with a large number of compounds. This further decreases the activation of endothelial lining of blood vessels. Finally, phytochemicals in muscadines have been shown to have profound beneficial effects on the behavior of macrophages and neutrophils and monocytes. These are processes involved in the inflammatory components of many disease states. Diets high in fruits and vegetables with anti-inflammatory phytochemicals can provide a "therapeutic reserve" in the treatment of multiple disease states. By therapeutic reserve, we mean that if drugs are needed above and beyond a well balanced anti-inflammatory diet, less drug will be needed to control the conditions. Above, we demonstrated that muscadine extract has significant anti-inflammatory power. Obviously, lower doses of pharmceutical agents such as aspirin, ibuprofen and naproxen may be necessary. Their power can be held in reserve for major crisis flare-ups. This is beneficial in that it reduces the side effects of higher doses of drugs. While many disease states call for additional drugs for other symptoms of the disease, the basic benefits of a diet enriched in anti-inflammatory phytochemicals can support many integrative medicine regimens. Muscadines, muscadine juice, wine, food supplements and nutraceutical products are sources of anti-inflammatory phytochemicals. Muscadines are a powerful choice for anti-inflammatory disease diets.

Readings For More Health Information

Eating Well for Optimal Health: The Essential Guide to Bringing Health and Pleasure Back to Eating by Andrew Weil

The Antioxidant Miracle by Lester Packer

Inflammation Nation by Floyd H. Chilton

Beyond Aspirin by Thomas M. Newmark and Paul Schulick

The Inflammation Syndrome by Jack Challem

The Omega Plan by Artemis P. Simopoulos and Jo Robinson

8 Weeks to Optimal Health by Andrew Weil

Dean Ornish's Program for Reversing Heart Disease by Dean Ornish

The 7 Day Color Diet by Weisel, Miller and Courtney

The Color Code: A Revolutionary Plan For Optimal Health by Underwood, Joseph and Nadeau

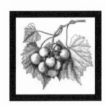

Chapter 8

Muscadines and Gastrointestinal Health

Muscadine Phytochemicals and Protection of the Oral Mucosa- There are several ways in which the phytochemicals in muscadines can protect the lining of the mouth, known as the oral muscosa. First, there are many antioxidant and anti-inflammatory compounds in muscadines. These have been described in Chapters 3 and 7. There are also antimicrobial, antiviral, antiseptic, anti-cariogenic, antiplaque and antigingivitis activities described for many of the phenolic substances in muscadines.

Oral Cancer- Oral precancerous lesions (leukoplakia) appear most frequently in tobacco smokers, but can occur in non-tobacco users as well. High fruit and vegetable intake has been associated with decreasing the rate of development of these lesions in tobacco users [436]. The incidence of developing these precancerous lesions is particularly high in smokeless tobacco users[437]. When you watch a baseball player with his chewing tobacco, think leukoplakia and oral cancer may be on its way. Teenagers are very susceptible to some of these fads, especially if they perceive the pros think it enhances athletic performance.

Anti-Oral Cancer Phytochemicals in Muscadines- Muscadine phyto-chemicals also have anti-oral cancer activities. Squamous cell carcinoma is a typical cancer of the mouth. Resveratrol or resveratrol in combination with quercetin inhibits the growth and DNA synthesis in an oral squamous cell tumor line. The effect was even greater if additional wine phytochemicals were added[438]. There appears to be considerable synergism or at least additivity among many of these grape phenolics. High ellagic acid extracts have been shown to prevent oral cancers in animal models [281, 439]. Muscadine skins and whole muscadine pomace extracts as nutraceutical products or as juice and wines may be highly protective against oral cancer due to the high ellagic acid content. There are probably many more phenolic substances in muscadine extracts that are equally as protective as those we have mentioned [440, 441]. Muscadine grape seeds share chemistry with grape seed extracts that are potent in killing two human oral tumor cell lines[442]. High proanthocyanidin grape seed extracts were significantly protective against smokeless tobacco-induced oxidative stress in human oral keratinocytes in culture[27]. Epidemiological studies have shown that chewing tobacco produces a very high risk of oral cancer[443]. Epidemiological studies consistently find that diets high in fruit consumption are protective against oral cancer [436, 444].

Muscadine Phytochemicals and Esophageal Protection- In general, the esophagus is subjected to a lot of wear and tear from swallowing boluses of rough or irritating food, drinking irritating liquids or swallowing irritating chemicals or drugs. Insofar as any of these produce injury, inflammation or oxidative stress, the highly anti-inflammatory and antioxidant compounds in muscadine grapes are surely beneficial. Muscadines contain a high concentration of ellagic acid and ellagic acid compounds in their skins, juice and seeds. Ellagic acid has been shown to be highly effective against esophageal cancers [285, 287, 289, 291, 293, 302, 303, 322, 325]. Any diet high in ellagic acid containing fruits is sure to be protective against carcinogenesis in the esophagus.

Adenocarcinoma of the esophagus has been increasing in incidence over the last 20 years in Western countries. There is a precancerous condition of the esophagus called Barrett's Esophagus that is often diagnosed in persons with chronic reflux of stomach contents into the esophagus. Since obesity tends to increase gastric reflux, and obesity rates are epidemic, there may be an association between obesity rates and the increase in esophageal cancer. There also may be diet related effects. COX-2 inhibitors are known to suppress bothe esophageal and large bowel cancer. Many flavonoids are powerful COX-2 inhibitors. Quercetin and ellagic acid have been shown to inhibit the growth of esophageal tumor cells. They do so by causing apoptosis, probably mediated by inhibition of NF-kappa B. In this regard, any of the substances in muscadine grapes that have been shown to be NF-kappa B inhibitors should contribute to the protection of the esophagus. See discussions of NF-kappa B in Chapters 4, 5, 6 and 7.

Protecting the Gastric Mucosa- Proanthocyanidins have been shown to protect the gastric muscosa under conditions of extreme experimental stress in rats[445]. They subjected rats to water-immersion restraint stress. This model produces stomach hemorrhagic ulcers in rats. If the rats had been taking proanthocyanidins in their drinking water, ulcer erosions were inhibited in a dose-dependent manner. They also found the mechanism involved anti-gastrin, anti-histamine effects while stimulating protective prostaglandin E2 and superoxide dismutase. These are important anti-ulcer activities.

Antioxidant phytochemicals can be highly protective of the stomach from oxidative free radical damage. They scavenge reactive nitrogen and oxygen species present in foods and preservatives. One interesting paper actually suggests that the stomach is a bioreactor and these oxidative free radicals can be absorbed and significantly impact the whole body. The presence of antioxidant phytochemicals in the diet makes a significant difference on what happens within the stomach[446]. Polyphenols can counteract prooxidant interactions catalyzed by metmyoglobin and/or iron ions. They showed that large increases in hydroperoxide concentration of oils or fats in meat in simulated gastric fluid

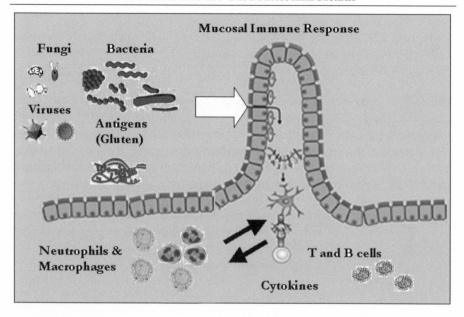

Figure 8.1. The immune system of the small intestine actively responds to bacteria, viruses, fungi and protein antigens. Cytokines are produced and immune cells move into the area. Muscadine phytochemicals permit the immune response to respond appropriately while suppressing development of chronic inflammation.

could be blocked by catechin and polyphenols. This certainly suggests that high flavonoid intake at meals is highly protective during the early digestive processes in the stomach. For a review of the many types of reactions taking place in the stomach that can produce free radicals see [447]. Heme proteins, lipid peroxides, aldehydes, isoprostance nitrites, chlorine species and hydrogen peroxides are a few of the substances that need to be dealt with by the stomach.

Protecting the Small Intestine- The same polyphenolics that the muscadine uses to protect itself from bacterial, viral or fungal attacks have anti-bacterial, anti-fungal and anti-viral properties inside humans also. These combinations may be particularly important in the gastrointestinal tract which is exposed to them in high concentrations. 60-70% of the immune system is sitting in the walls of the gut, waiting to defend us from "outsiders". The low pH of the stomach kills a lot of microorganisms, but when food moves into the small and large intestines, the pH is much higher and more favorable to bacterial growth. Protozoa are another sources of invaders that can significantly affect the condition of the gut wall. Any organism capable of aggravating the immune system sentinels in the wall of the gut, can set up a gut inflammation. The polyphenolic substances in muscadines are very potent anti-inflammatory agents and also have anti-bacterial, anti-fungal, anti-viral and anti-protozoal properties reported for them in the literature. In addition, muscadine extracts have tested to be very powerful anti-inflammatory fractions in both in vitro and in vivo tests [430]. This portends well for an anti-enteritis effect of muscadine products in the diet. See Figure 8.1 to understand the dual effects of anti-bacterial/anti-viral/anti-fungal activities with anti-inflammatory activities on immune cells in the walls of the intestine.

Muscadine Phytochemicals Defend Against Gastrointestinal Tract Cancers- Ellagic acid and its derivatives, gallic acid and its derivatives, the polyphenolics in general, resveratrol and its derivatives and a host of flavonoids are known to affect gastrointestinal health in many ways. Also, dietary fiber is known to affect gastrointestinal health. In summary, the muscadine grape is packed with phytochemicals that are good for the gastrointestinal system.

Flavonoids can have beneficial effects on the GI tract from the blood side when they are absorbed, but also may have benficial effects that are exerted directly within the GI tract. Many of these substances are only partially absorbed and so are in a position to affect the entire intestinal lining. The phenolic substances are known to bind prooxidant iron, scavenge nitrogen, chlorine and oxygen free radical species and many are known inhibitors of COX I and COX II and the lipoxygenases. [447]. That a high intake of flavonoids affects the entire GI tract has been verified by measuring the amount consumed and the amount of flavonoids and other phenols in human fecal contents.

Colon Cancer- In colon cancer or colorectal cancer, there is also thought to be a progression of abnormal cells that can eventually turn to cancer (Figure 6.1). The basic unit of the wall of the colon is called a crypt. Epithelial cells line these crypts. Stem cells are at the base of the crypt and they continuously proliferate to produce cells that divide and differentiate into the epithelial cells that line the surface of the inside of the colon. This process is very active because the cells lining the colon are sloughed off as lumenal contents move through the colon.

The first step in the initiation of colon cancer is a change in gene expression that disrupts the normal cell cycle and life. This change can occur due to mutation or epigenetic effects. Mutations are actually changes in DNA sequence that alters gene products. Epigenetic effects are due to genes being modified by methylation of the promotor region. Phytochemicals in the diet can affect both of these mechanisms and protect against colon cancer. Diet often brings mutagens to the colon in the form of chemicals formed in cooking food or meat. PhIP is one such mutagen. PhIP binds to DNA for form PhIP-DNA. This is called a DNA adduct and it keeps DNA from functioning properly. Flavonoid quercetin can block its formation of the DNA adduct in a dose-dependent manner. The same mutagen also produces liver cancer and its adducts to DNA can be prevented by phytochemicals [448-450].

Muscadine Phytochemicals Enhance the Effect of Beneficial Gut Flora-

High flavonoid diets are known to affect composition of gut flora [451]. While significant quantities of quercetin, myricetin and kaempferol are absorbed in the small intestine, a larger fraction of each remains in the lumen. Because flavonoids are rapidly converted to metabolites as they enter the blood, body cells are actually exposed to the derivatives. Gastrointestinal cells are exposed to a high concentration of flavonoids if they are in the diet. This leads to the probability that the work done in vitro with flavonoids may be very relevant to the in vivo situation. Flavonoids are known to suppress carcinogensis in multiple animal models. Their anti-cancer actions involve antioxidant activity and modulation of various cell signalling pathways that control cell cycle, cell differention and programmed cell death (apoptosis)[447].

Muscadine fiber was fed to hypercholesterolemic rats and it was shown that there were decreased amounts of fecal output of bile acids than in rats fed a comparable amount of bran [99,263]. Also, muscadine fiber has been compared with bran fibe. Fecal output and the levels of butyric acid in the cecum were increased in the muscadine-fed animals. These data indicated the muscadine fiber is a good bulking agent and is encouraging the production of the short chain fatty acids that are needed for good colon health[452] [96].

Colon health- Tartaric acid and fiber from raisins have also been shown to increase short chain fatty acid excretion and to lower the bile acid ratio of lithocholic to deoxylithocholic acid in humans[453, 454]. Short chain fatty acids are very necessary for providing a necessary energy source to colon cells. The presence of these in the stool suggests that the diet is encouraging production of these by the "good" bacteria needed in the colon for health. The bile acid ratio mentioned above is thought to correlate positively with a decrease risk of colon cancer in humans.

Once polyphenolics enter the colon, the can be extensively metabolized by colonic flora to generate different phenolics. Free radical scavenging, metal binding, and cell signalling modulation are each important actions that help to delay colon/rectal cancer development. In addition, many polyphenolics have actions to inhibit COX-2, LOX, angiogenesis, matrix metalloproteinases etc that are involved in cancer development. Is it any wonder that fruit and vegetable consumption is inversely associated with decreases in multiple types of cancers [455]? Vegetable and fruit consumption was found to be an independent indicator of decreased risk and was inversely related to mortality from cancer of the digestive tract. Fruit consumption was most highly correlated with this decrease risk[455]. Muscadines have the right profile of phytochemicals to be part of a healthy gastrointestinal system diet.

Chapter 9

Muscadines and Longevity

We think that the unique assortment of phytochemicals in muscadine grapes can help slow the effects of aging and possibly extend life. It is already known that smart dietary choices, risk avoidance, and useful physical activity can add ten years to life [456]. Evidence suggests that human populations should be able to live to an average age of about 85, which would mean that fewer people would be dying in their 50's and more would live to be 100. To maintain a good quality of life, it is important to prevent the loss of function or decline associated with old age. All the organs need to be conditioned, but it is particularly important to keep good mental function. Nothing shortens life faster than not being able to care for our loved ones and ourselves.

The first way to extend life was found to be reducing calorie intake while maintaining normal intakes of essential amino acids, fatty acids, vitamins and minerals [457-461]. The only problem with this approach is that the amount of life extension is most significant when food intake is restricted by at least one third. Calorie restricted animals have better immune function, less heart disease, fewer cancers, and longer life span, but they are hungry and not particularly happy campers. Who wants to give up good food just to live longer if it makes you miserable? This kind of life extension might work for animals in a cage but is unworkable for anyone who lives in the real world and has to work for a living. What we want is to be able to eat good food and still live longer.

Calorie Restriction, Gene Expression and Brain Aging
One of the ways to test how the body responds to a treatment is to analyze whether genes behave differently during the experiment. This has been done for calorie restricted animals. Animals that are fed normally have an increase in activity of stress-activated genes as they grow older. Calorie restriction tends to decrease the activity of the stress related genes [462-464]. This happens in just about every organ that has been tested, from muscle to liver to brain. So one of the theories of how calorie restriction extends life is that it helps protect the brain against age related injury. If nerve cells die, they usually can't be replaced, so it is very good news that we might be able to protect them. One of the theories is that aging increases oxidative stress and decreases our ability to combat it. Calorie restriction seems to boost the brains defenses while reducing the accumulation of tiny daily injuries.

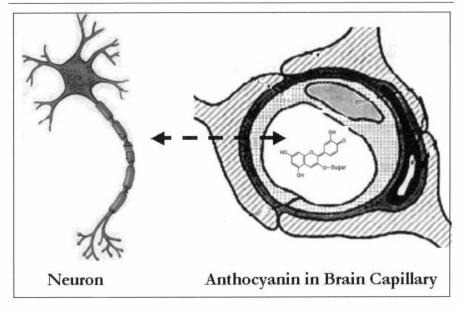

Neuron   **Anthocyanin in Brain Capillary**

Figure 9.1. Evidence shows that anthocyanins move from brain capillaries (right) across the blood-brain barrier (double arrow) into the brain, where they may stabilize nerve cells or neurons.

Berries, Leafy Greens and Brain Aging

If oxidative stress is part of what makes our brains age and part of what causes degenerative conditions like dementia and Alzheimer's disease, then perhaps the dietary antioxidants could help promote longevity. This idea has been tested extensively by providing high intakes of vitamin C, vitamin E and selenium. In general, the approach of increasing the essential antioxidants has not been very successful. One reason for this is that brain aging is not just due to oxygen free radicals. Inflammation, release of calcium from dying cells, and bleeding from tiny capillaries are other causes of brain aging. But there is good news. A dramatic breakthrough was found when animals were fed diets with extra blueberries, and in some cases, strawberries, spinach and kale have improved outcomes [465, 466].

One model used to test effects of berries and dark leafy greens is the Fischer 344 rat, which was developed expressly to study aging related disorders. When the animals age, their coordination and memory decline similarly to humans [467, 468]. The advantage of studying behavior in a dietary trial is that the animals can be tested for weeks and months. Psychologists have developed many kinds of tests such as the ability to get out of a maze, the ability to find food, and the ability to hang onto a rotating rod. Young animals remember details and quickly master these tasks, but older ones lose these abilities.

When animals were fed a diet that contained 1-2% dried blueberries, strawberries, or spinach, the blueberry fed animals maintained function significantly longer than animals that only got rodent chow [469]. The berries had the most beneficial effect, and when this news was reported in the popular press, the price of blueberries skyrocketed. Spinach also is protective, and grape seed extract rejuvenates brain antioxidant defenses [470].

Besides the fact that everyone is concerned about brain aging, there is something very interesting about these protective effects of some berries and leafy greens. The researchers believe that polyphenolics from the berries are probably responsible for providing extra protection, possibly by serving as powerful antioxidants. It is possible that phytochemicals could protect the brain through an indirect effect, but recent work shows that several of the anthocyanins do enter the brain [53, 471]. The anthocyanins are the red, blue and purple colored-phytochemicals in grapes. They are most abundant in dark colored grapes such as purple muscadine varieties. Other kinds of polyphenolics are not very well absorbed, and there is less evidence for beneficial effects on the brain. This topic is being studied very actively. There are plenty of anthocyanins in muscadine grapes, and many believe that "Anything blueberries can do, muscadines can do better!" They make better wine, too!

Plant Polyphenols and Antioxidant Defenses

Vitamins C, E, selenium and beta-carotene are all important dietary antioxidants. However, antioxidant defense is so important to the body that it makes its own powerful antioxidants. One of the most important is called glutathione, which is made of three amino acids linked together. One of the amino acids is cysteine, a sulfur amino acid that can be oxidized or reduced. Inside of cells, glutathione is kept in the reduced form so it can be an antioxidant. This is done by continually reducing any glutathione that gets oxidized using energy (actually electrons and protons) that are obtained from glucose.

It turns out that if glutathione is maintained at a high level, less vitamin C and E are needed. Now it has been shown that plant polyphenols such as quercetin and probably other flavonoids can increase the synthesis of glutathione in muscle and brain. This is good news because it means that small amounts of polyphenolics can improve antioxidant defenses indirectly. They appear to be activating a gene that encodes the enzyme that actually makes glutathione [472, 473] . The best defense against aging is definitely a good antioxidant defense. Muscadines have the right polyphenols to provide protection in all the ways we have discussed. Maybe muscadines and other berries are truly "brain foods." And most people like them a lot better than fish!

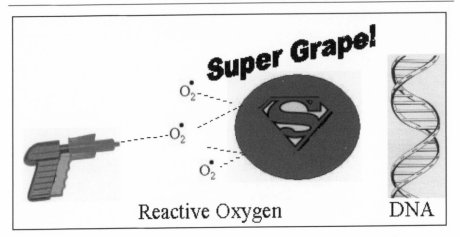

Figure 9.2. Daily metabolism produces free radicals that can damage DNA. Muscadine phytochemicals protect DNA against damage by eliminating free radicals, increasing glutathione defenses and enhancing the repair of DNA so mutations do not accumulate.

Resveratrol, Polyphenols and Life Extension

The effect of blueberries on brain function was definitely a step forward compared to calorie restriction, but it was just a first step. It turns out that overfeeding increases stress-associated genes in brain and other tissues, whereas consuming a highly nutritious diet that is restricted in calories decreases the activity of the stress associated genes [474, 475]. It has been known for years that calorie restriction increases lifespan. What has come as a surprise was the recent finding that plant polyphenols like resveratrol can also increase lifespan. There is hope for people who prefer to eat normal portions!

The discovery that polyphenolics including resveratrol and quercetin can extend lifespan was first made in yeast [476] and in a small worm that is used in aging studies because its genetics are well understood [477] . However, the same pathway is found in humans and it has already been shown that low concentrations of resveratrol activate a pathway that increases lifespan in human cells [476-478]. What happens is that a family of proteins called the sirtuins must be active in order for normal repair of DNA to occur, but the sirtuins are blocked (inhibited) by a chemical they produce called NAD [479]. When resveratrol or another plant phenolic is present, the sirtuins remain active. When they are active, DNA can be repaired and cells can live longer. Because DNA repair is improved, the cells do not collect mutations and become cancerous as rapidly as they do in the absence of resveratrol.

Activation of sirtuins has many other consequences that appear to be beneficial. One of their effects is to promote mobilization of fat from fat cells [480]. Another effect is to improve insulin sensitivity [481], and it is known that becoming fat decreases insulin sensitivity and raises blood glucose towards the diabetic range. The result is that muscadine grape chemicals including resveratrol, piceatannol and quercetin have many beneficial effects on our metabolism.

How to Benefit from Muscadine Polyphenols

The effects of plant polyphenols take place over the course of a few days and then wear off. The tests done with resveratrol and the sirtuins involve constant exposure to a low concentration (around 0.5 micromolar). Once the enzymes are active, their effects may persist for a day or two and then disappear, so it is best to plan meals to get several servings a week. A serving is about a cup of muscadine grapes or a cup of grape juice, or 6 ounces of wine. Yes, you can get these chemicals from other sources so the recommendation is to make sure your family is getting 5 or more servings a day of fruits, juices, berries, vegetables and whole grains. We believe that the 5-to-9 plan is sound, as long as one recognizes that muscadine grapes and certain berries have much more of the beneficial phytochemicals.

Plant Polyphenols and Chromosome Stability

One of the hallmarks of youth is that our chromosomes (which contain all of our genes) are full length and intact. As we get older, the chromosomes progressively shorten and eventually lose a protective cap on each end. The caps are called telomeres, and the ends get chewed off by an enzyme called telomerase. This is not a good thing, and it would be useful to block the enzyme so cells could continue dividing in a healthy manner.

Early tests concerning whether polyphenols affect the telomerase enzyme have been encouraging. The catechins in tea (especially green tea) do inhibit telomerase, and this has been suggested as one reason catechins have anti-cancer effects [482]. Muscadines also have catechins, and we are optimistic that muscadine extracts can be shown to inhibit telomerase. Estrogens activate telomerase, and there is potential for resveratrol to block this activation, but this has not yet been reported. There will soon be information about anthocyanins and other phytochemicals.

Take-Home Messages About Muscadines and Health

Earlier chapters in this book explain some of the beneficial effects of muscadine phytochemicals on the heart and blood vessels, how they defend against free radicals, reduce inflammatory diseases and may even prevent some cancers. People who eat foods that help defend their blood vessels and cardiovascular systems tend to stay healthy longer and not suffer from premature heart disease. Muscadine phytochemicals are good for the heart and blood vessels. Muscadines fit in well with a heart healthy diet, and that includes helping keep the blood pressure down, too. People who protect themselves from early heart disease and stroke are protecting themselves against conditions that account for nearly half of all deaths. One of the best rules for living a long time is, first, don't die young! Muscadines can help. One of the secrets to a long life is to pick healthy foods that actually taste good-like muscadines! Muscadine products can be among your powerful health choices!

Web Resources

Life Extension Foundation, http://www.lef.org/
Provides timely updates on aging research.

National Institute On Aging, http://www.nia.nih.gov/
The National Institute of Health that sponsors and evaluates peer-reviewed aging research

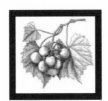

Chapter 10-

Muscadines and New Nutrition Science

Every health science changed on the day when the Human Genome project was completed, but not everyone understood why. In nutrition, the link is direct. Genes code for proteins, and the human genome encodes around 35,000 different proteins. Thousands of these genes are directly or indirectly responsible for nutrient metabolism. Some are enzymes that control glucose usage or fatty acid metabolism. Some are proteins that control gene expression, and these affect your health or are changed if your health becomes poor for any reason. Genes affect our heart health, blood vessel health, and immune health. Some genes protect against cancer, while others cause cancer. Genes are involved in blood glucose control, diabetes, and appetite control. They change during aging and in conditions such as osteoporosis and Alzheimer's disease. You name the disease, and genes are involved. But how are muscadines involved, and what benefit can they provide?

From about 1900-1950, most nutrition scientists studied essential nutrients that are needed for growth and maintenance of health. They were very focused on how to keep children and their parents healthy through the life cycle. The government got involved partly because it is a good thing if workers and soldiers report for duty in good health. Nutrients were seen as sources of energy (glucose, protein, and fats) or the vitamins and minerals needed to metabolize sources of energy and to build healthy bodies. As more was learned, the field of dietetics grew because of the need to counsel healthy people and hospital patients about the best available dietary advice.

Remarkably, the herbs and spices that add so much to great world cuisines had no place in nutrition texts of that era. Everyone knew they added flavors that make Chinese cuisine taste differently from Mediterranean dishes, Mexican foods or Thai meals. But no one really thought that spices might actually affect health. Similarly, people knew that the colors of foods were due to thousands of different phytochemicals, but very few of the colored compounds were known to affect our health (vitamin A and β-carotene were exceptions).

This perspective has totally changed because it is understood that genes directily respond to the food environment. It is true that spices are not used for energy and add no calories to a meal. But they (and muscadine phytonutrients) do affect gene expression and processes such as cell growth. Let us examine how.

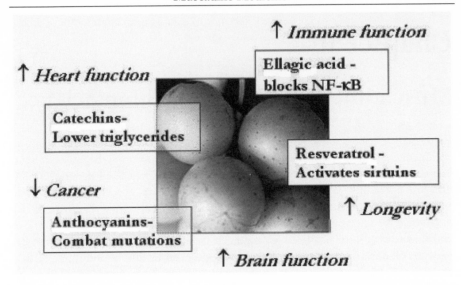

Figure 10.1. Purple and bronze muscadine grapes provide abundant phytochemicals that help maintain good health in all the ways shown, and more!

What you should know about genes and health- Most people do know that they inherit their genes from their parents. Many people may think that is all there is to it, and there is nothing you can do to modify gene function. Not so! Your diet and daily activities are the most powerful ways you can help your genes do what they need to do to keep you healthy. True, the number of genes you get will not change. But the activity of your genes is responsive to good nutrients, energy intake, sunshine, fresh air, healthy activity, and a good mood. Gene activity also responds to overeating, smog, refined foods, pollution, lack of activity, and feeling lousy! People who make good choices about their diets, family life, choices of occupation and leisure activities really are affecting their genes and their health. Let us examine a few cases in which muscadine phytonutrients affect genes in a good way. This is what we call the New Nutrition!

Muscadine nutrition and the genes of immune balance- Have you ever joked with a friend or family member about how many brain cells you have probably lost? We have-especially after one of those "senior moments" of forgetfulness! The fact is, no one looks in the mirror and says, "My body is made up of billions of cells so I should do what I can to protect them." But our bodies *are* made up of billions of cells and we really should do what we can for ourselves and our loved ones.

Figure 10.1 shows just a few of the phytonutrients in muscadines and scuppernongs and a few of their known actions on our health. Most people have never heard of these phytonutrients or the genes and biological processes they affect. Let us just say that the list is way too long to enumerate and it is growing daily!

The longer a person can maintain good immune function, the better are his chances of living a healthy life into the 80's and beyond. But if you think about arthritis for a moment, you know immunity is a double-edged sword. Yes, you want to be able to defend against infectious bacteria and viruses that make you sick. But if the immune system is over-active, it can make you unhealthy.

One of the proteins in the body that activates the immune system is called NF-κB. It starts a cascade that can get out of control. You want it to be somewhat active but not too active, and that is exactly what muscadine phytonutrients do. One of NF-κB's jobs is to respond to free radicals. Free radicals are oxidizing agents that turn on NF-κB the way you would turn on a light bulb in a dark room. But if you want a 100 watt bulb, you may not care for 1000 watts shining right in your eyes. Muscadine phytochemicals do not totally shut off NF-κB, they just turn it down.

NF-κB is a gene switch that is involved in all kinds of health problems. It tends to turn on genes that make hardening of the arteries and heart disease worse. It does the same thing for painful arthritis. It makes the HIV (AIDS) virus more active. It makes allergies and arthritis worse and increases the spread of cancers. Intestinal disorders like Crohn's disease flare up. Because NF-κB makes these problems worse, and phytochemicals turn down the heat, a diet that contains abundant phytochemicals can help people feel better. Muscadine chemicals probably can't completely cure these conditions, they just keep them from getting out of hand.

We all know some people who seem to age too soon, and others who sail along and never seem to show their age. Research has clearly shown that phytonutrients like the ones in muscadines and scuppernongs can help people live longer by up to 10 years with good life quality.

One of the most striking outcomes of the work with phytonutrients is that they really cut down on heart disease. Because men tend to get heart disease at a younger age than women, diets with lots of fruits, berries, vegetables and nuts help men live longer. The typical American male dies 5-7 years sooner than his wife, but the men who eat more phytonutrients live to almost the same age as their wives, on average, because the risk of cardiovascular disease drops. The gender difference in length of life drops to only 2 years in the lowest risk men [456].

Muscadine phytochemicals affect genes that keep every part of the body healthy- It is fairly easy to understand how phytonutrients in muscadine grapes can improve the health of the gastrointestinal tract. After all, eating grapes is a way of delivering these good chemicals to every part of the bowel. And it is not too hard to see how they could also affect the blood vessels to lower the

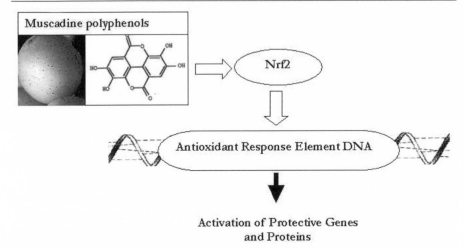

Activation of Protective Genes
and Proteins

Figure 10.2. Muscadine phytochemicals such as ellagic acid change gene activity. One example is the ability to activate a gene controller called Nrf2, which activates the Antioxidant Response Element in DNA. Activating this element activates production of a variety of proteins that protect cells against damage by free radicals.

incidence of heart disease. Once the phytonutrients are absorbed, they go into circulation in the blood, and some of them are carried on the same particles that move cholesterol around the body. Their antioxidant function prevents cholesterol from being even more damaging. But what about the tissues and organs that are a distance away from the site of absorption, such as the brain and the eyes, the prostate gland or the breasts?

More and more studies are showing that phytochemicals can reach all of these tissues and protect them. There are now ways to do sensitive tests on these tissues by looking at all the genes and proteins that are active. The tests are called gene expression tests or protein expression tests. Sometimes they are called gene array studies or proteomic studies. The point is that scientists are feeding animals diets that contain phytochemicals from muscadine grapes and other kinds of berries, fruits, and vegetables and looking for protection in these tissues. They are getting amazing results. One study provided diets to rats so that 5% of their calories were coming from grapes. Protein expression in the brain was studied, and the grape diet changed the expression of 17 different proteins in brain [184].

How do muscadine phytonutrients affect protective genes? Certain proteins act as master switches that activate many different proteins (Figure 10.2). Their job is to regulate our health and prevent damage. Just to give one example, there is a gene switch that turns on protective antioxidant enzymes and anti-cancer enzymes when there are too many free radicals or damaging chemicals in the area. The antioxidant response element (see figure above) is just one example of the many protective regulators that is affected by phytonutrients in muscadine grapes (and in broccoli and onions and other anti-cancer fruits and vegetables).

These master controllers are present in all of our vital organs. They are in the brain, heart, skin, liver and other vital organs. If your skin is exposed to too much sun, the burn you get is because of ultra-violet radiation. These damaging conditions activate the antioxidant response element, which tries to protect the skin. In this case, muscadine phytochemicals act almost like a sunscreen to add protection and help limit the damage. It is not just that the muscadine provides antioxidant protection (it does), but also that it is affecting protective genes.

Does this sound complicated? It is, but that is the new nutrition. Genetic switches such as NF-κB, the antioxidant response element and many others are affected by beneficial chemicals in phytochemical-rich foods like muscadines.

Muscadines and The New Science of Nutrition- Pick up any nutrition text that was written before 1990 and you might be surprised at what is not mentioned. Yes, you would find a list of all the essential vitamins, minerals, fatty acids, amino acids, carbohydrates and dietary fiber. You would find a discussion of how much energy is needed for work and sports, and some ideas about preventing obesity and diabetes and cancer. Add up all the essential nutrients, and you would have a list of maybe 50 compounds. Generations of nutritionists memorized these lists and learned to use computer programs to evaluate healthy diets. This is still done. So can you imagine how surprised even trained dietitians were to learn how many thousands of chemicals are in whole foods (but were never mentioned in the texts used at universities).

What was left out of traditional nutrition training in the United States until about the year 2000 was any appreciation that foods could do more than provide essential nutrients. Certainly anyone with an interest in cuisine knew that good food required special spices and sauces, and had flavors that are not found in carbohydrates, fats and proteins. No one knew that spices in cinnamon could lower blood glucose or that the turmeric in curries is an extremely powerful antioxidant. No one suspected that the chemicals that give whole foods, including muscadine grapes, their brilliant colors and intriguing tastes also improved a person's health.

The Take-Home Message- We should all provide whole, fresh foods like muscadine grapes in our families' diets. Not only does this plan provide energy, vitamins, and minerals, it also provides a range of phytochemicals that seem to give our genes a useful boost. Many phytochemicals are not traditional nutrients, but they alert our genes about how to prepare for and assimilate the nutrients in foods. They defend against free radicals and protect us by activating defensive systems that keep our cells parts intact, including the crucial DNA. We could not live without intact genes and DNA, so it is a good idea to work with it to keep it healthy.

The advice to eat 5 to 9 servings of fresh fruits and vegetables is very good and will not change any time soon. No one is suddenly going to say we should go back to high fat, overcooked, refined food. Not only should we be choosing 5 or more servings a day, we need to choose fruits and vegetables that have a lot of color and taste. The reason is that the new science of nutrition is showing that the phytochemicals that have the taste and color help protect our bodies from diseases. Traditional Southern foods like sweet potatoes, greens and muscadines all answer the call. And of course, we should chose other "power foods" including other fruits, berries, vegetables, crucifers, and legumes.

People who believe in taking dietary supplements and nutraceutical products do so because they are convenient, concentrated and alwarys on the shelf when the fresh fruit is not in season or if it just is not in the refrigerator today. Dietary supplements and nutraceutical products can add more phytochemical insurance to diets that vary from day to day. Finally, as we battle a worldwide epidemic of obesity, diabetes and metabolic syndrome, food restriction in the context of a healthy diet is important. Food supplements and nutraceutical products add phytochemical power without adding unnecessary calories.

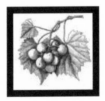

A TOAST To The MUSCADINE INDUSTRY !

The authors propose a toast to the American grapevine, *Vitis rotundifolia,* and the people who bring fine muscadine products to the world!

~To Health!~

Biomedical References

1.   Ulmer M, Beck SE: **Cherokee Cooklore. To Make My Bread.** Cherokee, N.C.: Museum of the Cherokee Indian; 1951.
2.   Gohdes C: **Scuppernong, North Carolina's Grape and Its Wines**. Durham, NC: Duke University Press; 1982.
3.   Baek HH, Cadwallader KR, Marroquin E, Silva JL: **Identification of predominant aroma compounds in muscadine grape juice**. *Journal of Food Science* 1997, **62**(2):249-252.
4.   Lamikanra O: **Aroma Constituents of Muscadine Wines**. *Journal of Food Quality* 1987, **10**(1):57-66.
5.   Lee JH, Talcott ST: **Ellagic acid and ellagitannins affect on sedimentation in muscadine juice and wine**. *J Agric Food Chem* 2002, **50**(14):3971-3976.
6.   DeFelice SL: **The NutraCeutical Revolution: Fueling a Powerful, New International Market**. In: *Harvard University Advanced Program in Biomedical Research Management and Development: 1986; Como, Italy*; 1986.
7.   Viljoen TA, JJ S: **Cytogenetical studies of three Vitis species**. *Vitis* 1970, **34**((4)):221-224.
8.   Patel GI, Olmo HP: **Cytogenetics of Vitis. I. The hybrid V. vinifera times V. rotundifolia**. *Amer J Botany* 1955, **42**:141-155.
9.   Ector BJ, Welch AS, Harkness E, Hegwood CP: **Nutritional components of red muscadine grapes: Levels of protein, carbohydrate, fat, dietary fiber, pectin and selected minerals and vitamins**. In: *Southern Assoc Agric Scientists, Food Sci Human Nutr Sec: 1993*; 1993: 32.
10.   Silva JL, Garner JO, Woods F, Ghaedian R: **Physicochemical and sensory properties of muscadine grape**. *Journal of Food Quality* 1993, **16**(2):81-90.
11.   Boyle JA, Hsu L: **Identification and Quantitation of Ellagic Acid in Muscadine Grape Juice**. *American Journal of Enology and Viticulture* 1990, **41**(1):43-47.
12.   Nowson CA, Worsley A, Margerison C, Jorna MK, Godfrey SJ, Booth A: **Blood pressure change with weight loss is affected by diet type in men**. *Am J Clin Nutr* 2005, **81**(5):983-989.
13.   Most MM: **Estimated phytochemical content of the dietary approaches to stop hypertension (DASH) diet is higher than in the Control Study Diet**. *J Am Diet Assoc* 2004, **104**(11):1725-1727.
14.   **Can blood pressure be lowered by a change in diet? Evidence from the DASH trials**. *Can Fam Physician* 2004, **50**:375.
15.   Doyle L, Cashman KD: **The DASH diet may have beneficial effects on bone health**. *Nutr Rev* 2004, **62**(5):215-220.
16.   Booth AO, Nowsen CA, Worsley T, Margerison C, Jorna MK: **Dietary approaches for weight loss with increased fruit, vegetables and dairy**. *Asia Pac J Clin Nutr* 2003, **12** Suppl:S10.
17.   He FJ, MacGregor GA: **Potassium: more beneficial effects**. *Climacteric* 2003, **6 Suppl 3**:36-48.
18.   Lopes HF, Martin KL, Nashar K, Morrow JD, Goodfriend TL, Egan BM: **DASH diet lowers blood pressure and lipid-induced oxidative stress in obesity**. *Hypertension* 2003, **41**(3):422-430.
19.   Davy BM, Melby CL: **The effect of fiber-rich carbohydrates on features of Syndrome X**. *J Am Diet Assoc* 2003, **103**(1):86-96.
20.   Blackburn GL: **Salt shakedown. DASH diet beats salt restriction at lowering blood pressure**. *Health News* 2002, **8**(12):5.
21.   Bagchi D, Sen CK, Ray SD, Das DK, Bagchi M, Preuss HG, Vinson JA: **Molecular mechanisms of cardioprotection by a novel grape seed proanthocyanidin extract**. *Mutat Res* 2003, **523-524**:87-97.

22. Bagchi D, Ray SD, Bagchi M, Preuss HG, Stohs SJ: **Mechanistic pathways of antioxidant cytoprotection by a novel IH636 grape seed proanthocyanidin extract.** *Indian J Exp Biol* 2002, **40**(6):717-726.

23. Vinson JA, Mandarano MA, Shuta DL, Bagchi M, Bagchi D: **Beneficial effects of a novel IH636 grape seed proanthocyanidin extract and a niacin-bound chromium in a hamster atherosclerosis model.** *Mol Cell Biochem* 2002, **240**(1-2):99-103.

24. Bagchi D, Bagchi M, Stohs S, Ray SD, Sen CK, Preuss HG: **Cellular protection with proanthocyanidins derived from grape seeds.** *Ann N Y Acad Sci* 2002, **957**:260-270.

25. Wren AF, Cleary M, Frantz C, Melton S, Norris L: **90-day oral toxicity study of a grape seed extract (IH636) in rats.** *J Agric Food Chem* 2002, **50**(7):2180-2192.

26. Ray S, Bagchi D, Lim PM, Bagchi M, Gross SM, Kothari SC, Preuss HG, Stohs SJ: **Acute and long-term safety evaluation of a novel IH636 grape seed proanthocyanidin extract.** *Res Commun Mol Pathol Pharmacol* 2001, **109**(3-4):165-197.

27. Bagchi M, Kuszynski CA, Balmoori J, Joshi SS, Stohs SJ, Bagchi D: **Protective effects of antioxidants against smokeless tobacco-induced oxidative stress and modulation of Bcl-2 and p53 genes in human oral keratinocytes.** *Free Radic Res* 2001, **35**(2):181-194.

28. Banerjee B, Bagchi D: **Beneficial effects of a novel IH636 grape seed proanthocyanidin extract in the treatment of chronic pancreatitis.** *Digestion* 2001, **63**(3):203-206.

29. Ray SD, Patel D, Wong V, Bagchi D: **In vivo protection of dna damage associated apoptotic and necrotic cell deaths during acetaminophen-induced nephrotoxicity, amiodarone-induced lung toxicity and doxorubicin-induced cardiotoxicity by a novel IH636 grape seed proanthocyanidin extract.** *Res Commun Mol Pathol Pharmacol* 2000, **107**(1-2):137-166.

30. Ray SD, Wong V, Rinkovsky A, Bagchi M, Raje RR, Bagchi D: **Unique organoprotective properties of a novel IH636 grape seed proanthocyanidin extract on cadmium chloride-induced nephrotoxicity, dimethylnitrosamine (DMN)-induced splenotoxicity and mocap-induced neurotoxicity in mice.** *Res Commun Mol Pathol Pharmacol* 2000, **107**(1-2):105-128.

31. Ray SD, Parikh H, Hickey E, Bagchi M, Bagchi D: **Differential effects of IH636 grape seed proanthocyanidin extract and a DNA repair modulator 4-aminobenzamide on liver microsomal cytochrome 4502E1-dependent aniline hydroxylation.** *Mol Cell Biochem* 2001, **218**(1-2):27-33.

32. Bagchi D, Ray SD, Patel D, Bagchi M: **Protection against drug- and chemical-induced multiorgan toxicity by a novel IH636 grape seed proanthocyanidin extract.** *Drugs Exp Clin Res* 2001, **27**(1):3-15.

33. Joshi SS, Kuszynski CA, Benner EJ, Bagchi M, Bagchi D: **Amelioration of the cytotoxic effects of chemotherapeutic agents by grape seed proanthocyanidin extract.** *Antioxid Redox Signal* 1999, **1**(4):563-570.

34. Bagchi D, Bagchi M, Stohs SJ, Das DK, Ray SD, Kuszynski CA, Joshi SS, Pruess HG: **Free radicals and grape seed proanthocyanidin extract: importance in human health and disease prevention.** *Toxicology* 2000, **148**(2-3):187-197.

35. Ray SD, Kumar MA, Bagchi D: **A novel proanthocyanidin IH636 grape seed extract increases in vivo Bcl-XL expression and prevents acetaminophen-induced programmed and unprogrammed cell death in mouse liver.** *Arch Biochem Biophys* 1999, **369**(1):42-58.

36. Ye X, Krohn RL, Liu W, Joshi SS, Kuszynski CA, McGinn TR, Bagchi M, Preuss HG, Stohs SJ, Bagchi D: **The cytotoxic effects of a novel IH636 grape seed proanthocyanidin extract on cultured human cancer cells.** *Mol Cell Biochem* 1999, **196**(1-2):99-108.

37. Bagchi M, Balmoori J, Bagchi D, Ray SD, Kuszynski C, Stohs SJ: **Smokeless tobacco, oxidative stress, apoptosis, and antioxidants in human oral keratinocytes.** *Free Radic Biol Med* 1999, **26**(7-8):992-1000.

38. Wu X, Beecher GR, Holden JM, Haytowitz DB, Gebhardt SE, Prior RL: **Lipophilic and hydrophilic antioxidant capacities of common foods in the United States.** *J Agric Food Chem* 2004, **52**(12):4026-4037.

39. Proteggente AR, Pannala AS, Paganga G, Van Buren L, Wagner E, Wiseman S, Van De Put F, Dacombe C, Rice-Evans CA: **The antioxidant activity of regularly consumed fruit and vegetables reflects their phenolic and vitamin C composition.** *Free Radic Res* 2002, **36**(2):217-233.

40. Wang H, Cao GH, Prior RL: **Total antioxidant capacity of fruits.** *Journal of Agricultural and Food Chemistry* 1996, **44**(3):701-705.

41. Ehlenfeldt MK, Prior RL: **Oxygen radical absorbance capacity (ORAC) and phenolic and anthocyanin concentrations in fruit and leaf tissues of highbush blueberry.** *J Agric Food Chem* 2001, **49**(5):2222-2227.

42. Cho MJ, Howard LR, Prior RL, Clark JR: **Flavonoid glycosides and antioxidant capacity of varous blackberry, blueberry and red grape genotypes determined by high-performance liquid chromatography/mass spectrometry.** *Journal of the Science of Food and Agriculture* 2004, **84**(13):1771-1782.

43. Talcott ST, Lee JH: **Ellagic acid and flavonoid antioxidant content of muscadine wine and juice.** *J Agric Food Chem* 2002, **50**(11):3186-3192.

44. Morris JR, Brady PL: **The Muscadine Experience. Adding Value to Enhance Profits.** *Arkansas Agricultural Experiment Station Research Reports* 2004, **974**:1-80.

45. Klatsky AL, Friedman GD, Armstrong MA, Kipp H: **Wine, liquor, beer, and mortality.** *Am J Epidemiol* 2003, **158**(6):585-595.

46. Bruneton J: **Pharmacognosy. Phytochemistry. Medicinal Plants,** 2nd edn. Paris: Lavoisier Publishing; 1999.

47. Polya GM: **Biochemical targets of plant bioactive compounds : a pharmacological reference guide to sites of action and biological effects.** New York: Taylor & Francis; 2003.

48. Meskin MS, Bidlack WR, Davies AJ, Lewis DS, Randolph RK: **Phytochemicals. Mechanisms of Action.** Boca Raton: CRC Press; 2004.

49. Williamson G: **Common Features in the Pathways of Absorption and Metabolism of Flavonoids.** In: *Phytochemicals Mechanisms of Action.* Edited by Mark S. Meskin WRB, Audra J. Davies, Douglas S. Lewis, R. Keith Randolph. Boca Raton: CRC Press LLC; 2004: 21-34.

50. Prior RL: **Absorption and Metabolism of Anthocyanins: Potential Health Effects.** In: *Phytochemicals: Mechanisms of Action.* Edited by Meskin MS, Bidlack, W.R., Davies, A.J., Lewis, D.S. and Randolph, R.K. Boca Raton: CRC Press; 2004: 1-19.

51. Day AJ, Mellon F, Barron D, Sarrazin G, Morgan MR, Williamson G: **Human metabolism of dietary flavonoids: identification of plasma metabolites of quercetin.** *Free Radic Res* 2001, **35**(6):941-952.

52. Galli RL, Bielinski DF, Szprengiel A, Shukitt-Hale B, Joseph JA: **Blueberry supplemented diet reverses age-related decline in hippocampal HSP70 neuroprotection.** *Neurobiol Aging* 2005.

53. Galli RL, Shukitt-Hale B, Youdim KA, Joseph JA: **Fruit polyphenolics and brain aging: nutritional interventions targeting age-related neuronal and behavioral deficits.** *Ann N Y Acad Sci* 2002, **959**:128-132.

54. Koh HH, Murray IJ, Nolan D, Carden D, Feather J, Beatty S: **Plasma and macular responses to lutein supplement in subjects with and without age-related maculopathy: a pilot study.** *Exp Eye Res* 2004, **79**(1):21-27.

55. Youdim KA, Martin A, Joseph JA: **Incorporation of the elderberry anthocyanins by endothelial cells increases protection against oxidative stress.** *Free Radic Biol Med* 2000, **29**(1):51-60.

56. Kammerer D, Claus A, Carle R, Schieber A: **Polyphenol screening of pomace from red and white grape varieties (Vitis vinifera L.) by HPLC-DAD-MS/MS.** *J Agric Food Chem* 2004, **52**(14):4360-4367.

57. Lee JH, Johnson JV, Talcott ST: **Identification of ellagic acid conjugates and other polyphenolics in muscadine grapes by HPLC-ESI-MS.** *J Agric Food Chem* 2005, **53**(15):6003-6010.

58. Wu X, Cao G, Prior RL: **Absorption and metabolism of anthocyanins in elderly women after consumption of elderberry or blueberry.** *J Nutr* 2002, **132**(7):1865-1871.

59. Cao G, Muccitelli HU, Sanchez-Moreno C, Prior RL: **Anthocyanins are absorbed in glycated forms in elderly women: a pharmacokinetic study.** *Am J Clin Nutr* 2001, **73**(5):920-926.

60. Matsumoto H, Inaba H, Kishi M, Tominaga S, Hirayama M, Tsuda T: **Orally administered delphinidin 3-rutinoside and cyanidin 3-rutinoside are directly absorbed in rats and humans and appear in the blood as the intact forms.** *J Agric Food Chem* 2001, **49**(3):1546-1551.

61. Miyazawa T, Nakagawa K, Kudo M, Muraishi K, Someya K: **Direct intestinal absorption of red fruit anthocyanins, cyanidin-3-glucoside and cyanidin-3,5-diglucoside, into rats and humans.** *J Agric Food Chem* 1999, **47**(3):1083-1091.

62. Prior RL: **Fruits and vegetables in the prevention of cellular oxidative damage.** *Am J Clin Nutr* 2003, **78**(3 Suppl):570S-578S.

63. Romero-Perez AI, Ibern-Gomez M, Lamuela-Raventos RM, de La Torre-Boronat MC: **Piceid, the major resveratrol derivative in grape juices.** *J Agric Food Chem* 1999, **47**(4):1533-1536.

64. Sato M, Suzuki Y, Okuda T, Yokotsuka K: **Contents of resveratrol, piceid, and their isomers in commercially available wines made from grapes cultivated in Japan.** *Biosci Biotechnol Biochem* 1997, **61**(11):1800-1805.

65. Hollman PC, de Vries JH, van Leeuwen SD, Mengelers MJ, Katan MB: **Absorption of dietary quercetin glycosides and quercetin in healthy ileostomy volunteers.** *Am J Clin Nutr* 1995, **62**(6):1276-1282.

66. Paganga G, Rice-Evans CA: **The identification of flavonoids as glycosides in human plasma.** *FEBS Lett* 1997, **401**(1):78-82.

67. Rimando AM, Nagmani R, Feller DR, Yokoyama W: **Pterostilbene, a new agonist for the peroxisome proliferator-activated receptor alpha-isoform, lowers plasma lipoproteins and cholesterol in hypercholesterolemic hamsters.** *J Agric Food Chem* 2005, **53**(9):3403-3407.

68. Stoclet JC, Chataigneau T, Ndiaye M, Oak MH, El Bedoui J, Chataigneau M, Schini-Kerth VB: **Vascular protection by dietary polyphenols.** *Eur J Pharmacol* 2004, **500**(1-3):299-313.

69. Gonzalez-Gay MA, Gonzalez-Juanatey C, Martin J: **Rheumatoid arthritis: a disease associated with accelerated atherogenesis.** *Semin Arthritis Rheum* 2005, **35**(1):8-17.

70. Thuillez C, Richard V: **Targeting endothelial dysfunction in hypertensive subjects.** *J Hum Hypertens* 2005, **19 Suppl 1**:S21-25.

71. Wilson KM, Lentz SR: **Mechanisms of the atherogenic effects of elevated homocysteine in experimental models.** *Semin Vasc Med* 2005, **5**(2):163-171.

72. Costacou T, Lopes-Virella MF, Zgibor JC, Virella G, Otvos J, Walsh M, Orchard TJ: **Markers of endothelial dysfunction in the prediction of coronary artery disease in Type 1 diabetes. The Pittsburgh Epidemiology of Diabetes Complications Study.** *J Diabetes Complications* 2005, **19**(4):183-193.

73. Avogaro A, de Kreutzenberg SV: **Mechanisms of endothelial dysfunction in obesity.** *Clin Chim Acta* 2005.

74. Hink U, Tsilimingas N, Wendt M, Munzel T: **Mechanisms underlying endothelial dysfunction in diabetes mellitus: therapeutic implications.** *Treat Endocrinol* 2003, **2**(5):293-304.

75. Frein D, Schildknecht S, Bachschmid M, Ullrich V: **Redox regulation: A new challenge for pharmacology.** *Biochem Pharmacol* 2005.

76. Fortuno A, Jose GS, Moreno MU, Diez J, Zalba G: **Oxidative stress and vascular remodelling.** *Exp Physiol* 2005, **90**(4):457-462.

77. Hertog MG, Kromhout D, Aravanis C, Blackburn H, Buzina R, Fidanza F, Giampaoli S, Jansen A, Menotti A, Nedeljkovic S *et al*: **Flavonoid intake and long-term risk of**

coronary heart disease and cancer in the seven countries study. *Arch Intern Med* 1995, **155**(4):381-386.

78. Hertog MG, Feskens EJ, Hollman PC, Katan MB, Kromhout D: **Dietary antioxidant flavonoids and risk of coronary heart disease: the Zutphen Elderly Study.** *Lancet* 1993, **342**(8878):1007-1011.

79. Hertog MG, Feskens EJ, Hollman PC, Katan MB, Kromhout D: **Dietary flavonoids and cancer risk in the Zutphen Elderly Study.** *Nutr Cancer* 1994, **22**(2):175-184.

80. Hertog MG, Hollman PC: **Potential health effects of the dietary flavonol quercetin.** *Eur J Clin Nutr* 1996, **50**(2):63-71.

81. German JB, Walzem RL: **The health benefits of wine.** *Annu Rev Nutr* 2000, **20**:561-593.

82. Goldberg IJ, Mosca L, Piano MR, Fisher EA: **AHA Science Advisory: Wine and your heart: a science advisory for healthcare professionals from the Nutrition Committee, Council on Epidemiology and Prevention, and Council on Cardiovascular Nursing of the American Heart Association.** *Circulation* 2001, **103**(3):472-475.

83. Renaud S, de Lorgeril M: **Wine, alcohol, platelets, and the French paradox for coronary heart disease.** *Lancet* 1992, **339**(8808):1523-1526.

84. Brown AJ, Leong SL, Dean RT, Jessup W: **7-Hydroperoxycholesterol and its products in oxidized low density lipoprotein and human atherosclerotic plaque.** *J Lipid Res* 1997, **38**(9):1730-1745.

85. Lynch SM, Morrow JD, Roberts LJ, 2nd, Frei B: **Formation of non-cyclooxygenase-derived prostanoids (F2-isoprostanes) in plasma and low density lipoprotein exposed to oxidative stress in vitro.** *J Clin Invest* 1994, **93**(3):998-1004.

86. Mangiapane H, Thomson J, Salter A, Brown S, Bell GD, White DA: **The inhibition of the oxidation of low density lipoprotein by (+)-catechin, a naturally occurring flavonoid.** *Biochem Pharmacol* 1992, **43**(3):445-450.

87. Brown JE, Khodr H, Hider RC, Rice-Evans CA: **Structural dependence of flavonoid interactions with Cu2+ ions: implications for their antioxidant properties.** *Biochem J* 1998, **330** (**Pt 3**):1173-1178.

88. de Whalley CV, Rankin SM, Hoult JR, Jessup W, Leake DS: **Flavonoids inhibit the oxidative modification of low density lipoproteins by macrophages.** *Biochem Pharmacol* 1990, **39**(11):1743-1750.

89. Chou EJ, Keevil JG, Aeschlimann S, Wiebe DA, Folts JD, Stein JH: **Effect of ingestion of purple grape juice on endothelial function in patients with coronary heart disease.** *Am J Cardiol* 2001, **88**(5):553-555.

90. Stein JH, Keevil JG, Wiebe DA, Aeschlimann S, Folts JD: **Purple grape juice improves endothelial function and reduces the susceptibility of LDL cholesterol to oxidation in patients with coronary artery disease.** *Circulation* 1999, **100**(10):1050-1055.

91. Aviram M: **The contribution of the macrophage receptor for oxidized LDL to its cellular uptake.** *Biochem Biophys Res Commun* 1991, **179**(1):359-365.

92. Maor I, Kaplan M, Hayek T, Vaya J, Hoffman A, Aviram M: **Oxidized monocyte-derived macrophages in aortic atherosclerotic lesion from apolipoprotein E-deficient mice and from human carotid artery contain lipid peroxides and oxysterols.** *Biochem Biophys Res Commun* 2000, **269**(3):775-780.

93. Achike FI, Kwan CY: **Nitric oxide, human diseases and the herbal products that affect the nitric oxide signalling pathway.** *Clin Exp Pharmacol Physiol* 2003, **30**(9):605-615.

94. Dell'Agli M, Galli GV, Vrhovsek U, Mattivi F, Bosisio E: **In vitro inhibition of human cGMP-specific phosphodiesterase-5 by polyphenols from red grapes.** *J Agric Food Chem* 2005, **53**(6):1960-1965.

95. Gupta M, Kovar A, Meibohm B: **The clinical pharmacokinetics of phosphodiesterase-5 inhibitors for erectile dysfunction.** *J Clin Pharmacol* 2005, **45**(9):987-1003.

96. Ector BJ: **Compositional and Nutritional Characteristics.** In: *Muscadine Grapes.* Edited by Basiouny FMaH, D.G. Alexandria, VA: ASHS Press; 2001.

97.   Abe I, Kashiwagi Y, Noguchi H, Tanaka T, Ikeshiro Y, Kashiwada Y: **Ellagitannins and hexahydroxydiphenoyl esters as inhibitors of vertebrate squalene epoxidase.** *J Nat Prod* 2001, **64**(8):1010-1014.

98.   Folts JD: **Potential health benefits from the flavonoids in grape products on vascular disease.** *Adv Exp Med Biol* 2002, **505**:95-111.

99.   Knekt P, Kumpulainen J, Jarvinen R, Rissanen H, Heliovaara M, Reunanen A, Hakulinen T, Aromaa A: **Flavonoid intake and risk of chronic diseases.** *Am J Clin Nutr* 2002, **76**(3):560-568.

100. Geleijnse JM, Launer LJ, Van der Kuip DA, Hofman A, Witteman JC: **Inverse association of tea and flavonoid intakes with incident myocardial infarction: the Rotterdam Study.** *Am J Clin Nutr* 2002, **75**(5):880-886.

101. Arai Y, Watanabe S, Kimira M, Shimoi K, Mochizuki R, Kinae N: **Dietary intakes of flavonols, flavones and isoflavones by Japanese women and the inverse correlation between quercetin intake and plasma LDL cholesterol concentration.** *J Nutr* 2000, **130**(9):2243-2250.

102. Rendig SV, Symons JD, Longhurst JC, Amsterdam EA: **Effects of red wine, alcohol, and quercetin on coronary resistance and conductance arteries.** *J Cardiovasc Pharmacol* 2001, **38**(2):219-227.

103. Abou-Agag LH, Aikens ML, Tabengwa EM, Benza RL, Shows SR, Grenett HE, Booyse FM: **Polyphyenolics increase t-PA and u-PA gene transcription in cultured human endothelial cells.** *Alcohol Clin Exp Res* 2001, **25**(2):155-162.

104. Di Santo A, Mezzetti A, Napoleone E, Di Tommaso R, Donati MB, De Gaetano G, Lorenzet R: **Resveratrol and quercetin down-regulate tissue factor expression by human stimulated vascular cells.** *J Thromb Haemost* 2003, **1**(5):1089-1095.

105. Chan MM, Mattiacci JA, Hwang HS, Shah A, Fong D: **Synergy between ethanol and grape polyphenols, quercetin, and resveratrol, in the inhibition of the inducible nitric oxide synthase pathway.** *Biochem Pharmacol* 2000, **60**(10):1539-1548.

106. Kaneider NC, Mosheimer B, Reinisch N, Patsch JR, Wiedermann CJ: **Inhibition of thrombin-induced signaling by resveratrol and quercetin: effects on adenosine nucleotide metabolism in endothelial cells and platelet-neutrophil interactions.** *Thromb Res* 2004, **114**(3):185-194.

107. Hubbard GP, Wolffram S, Lovegrove JA, Gibbins JM: **The role of polyphenolic compounds in the diet as inhibitors of platelet function.** *Proc Nutr Soc* 2003, **62**(2):469-478.

108. Mardla V, Kobzar G, Samel N: **Potentiation of antiaggregating effect of prostaglandins by alpha-tocopherol and quercetin.** *Platelets* 2004, **15**(5):319-324.

109. Hubbard GP, Wolffram S, Lovegrove JA, Gibbins JM: **Ingestion of quercetin inhibits platelet aggregation and essential components of the collagen-stimulated platelet activation pathway in humans.** *J Thromb Haemost* 2004, **2**(12):2138-2145.

110. Brookes PS, Digerness SB, Parks DA, Darley-Usmar V: **Mitochondrial function in response to cardiac ischemia-reperfusion after oral treatment with quercetin.** *Free Radic Biol Med* 2002, **32**(11):1220-1228.

111. Soloviev A, Stefanov A, Parshikov A, Khromov A, Moibenko A, Kvotchina L, Balavoine G, Geletii Y: **Arrhythmogenic peroxynitrite-induced alterations in mammalian heart contractility and its prevention with quercetin-filled liposomes.** *Cardiovasc Toxicol* 2002, **2**(2):129-139.

112. Qin TC, Chen L, Yu LX, Gu ZL: **Inhibitory effect of quercetin on cultured neonatal rat cardiomyocytes hypertrophy induced by angiotensin.** *Acta Pharmacol Sin* 2001, **22**(12):1103-1106.

113. Ruf JC: **Alcohol, wine and platelet function.** *Biol Res* 2004, **37**(2):209-215.

114. Ruf JC: **Wine and polyphenols related to platelet aggregation and atherothrombosis.** *Drugs Exp Clin Res* 1999, **25**(2-3):125-131.

115. Wu JM, Wang ZR, Hsieh TC, Bruder JL, Zou JG, Huang YZ: **Mechanism of cardioprotection by resveratrol, a phenolic antioxidant present in red wine (Review).** *Int J Mol Med* 2001, **8**(1):3-17.

116. Wang Z, Huang Y, Zou J, Cao K, Xu Y, Wu JM: **Effects of red wine and wine polyphenol resveratrol on platelet aggregation in vivo and in vitro.** *Int J Mol Med* 2002, **9**(1):77-79.

117. Zou JG, Wang ZR, Huang YZ, Cao KJ, Wu JM: **Effect of red wine and wine polyphenol resveratrol on endothelial function in hypercholesterolemic rabbits.** *Int J Mol Med* 2003, **11**(3):317-320.

118. Bhat KPL, Kosmeder JW, 2nd, Pezzuto JM: **Biological effects of resveratrol.** *Antioxid Redox Signal* 2001, **3**(6):1041-1064.

119. Bradamante S, Barenghi L, Villa A: **Cardiovascular protective effects of resveratrol.** *Cardiovasc Drug Rev* 2004, **22**(3):169-188.

120. Fremont L: **Biological effects of resveratrol.** *Life Sci* 2000, **66**(8):663-673.

121. Asou H, Koshizuka K, Kyo T, Takata N, Kamada N, Koeffier HP: **Resveratrol, a natural product derived from grapes, is a new inducer of differentiation in human myeloid leukemias.** *Int J Hematol* 2002, **75**(5):528-533.

122. Ferrero ME, Bertelli AE, Fulgenzi A, Pellegatta F, Corsi MM, Bonfrate M, Ferrara F, De Caterina R, Giovannini L, Bertelli A: **Activity in vitro of resveratrol on granulocyte and monocyte adhesion to endothelium.** *Am J Clin Nutr* 1998, **68**(6):1208-1214.

123. Carluccio MA, Siculella L, Ancora MA, Massaro M, Scoditti E, Storelli C, Visioli F, Distante A, De Caterina R: **Olive oil and red wine antioxidant polyphenols inhibit endothelial activation: antiatherogenic properties of Mediterranean diet phytochemicals.** *Arterioscler Thromb Vasc Biol* 2003, **23**(4):622-629.

124. Bertelli AA, Baccalini R, Battaglia E, Falchi M, Ferrero ME: **Resveratrol inhibits TNF alpha-induced endothelial cell activation.** *Therapie* 2001, **56**(5):613-616.

125. Ahn KS, Kim JH, Oh SR, Ryu SY, Lee HK: **Inhibitory activity of stilbenes from medicinal plants on the expression of cell adhesion molecules on THP1 cells.** *Planta Med* 2000, **66**(7):641-644.

126. de la Lastra CA, Villegas I: **Resveratrol as an anti-inflammatory and anti-aging agent: mechanisms and clinical implications.** *Mol Nutr Food Res* 2005, **49**(5):405-430.

127. Elmali N, Esenkaya I, Harma A, Ertem K, Turkoz Y, Mizrak B: **Effect of resveratrol in experimental osteoarthritis in rabbits.** *Inflamm Res* 2005, **54**(4):158-162.

128. Leiro J, Arranz JA, Fraiz N, Sanmartin ML, Quezada E, Orallo F: **Effect of cis-resveratrol on genes involved in nuclear factor kappa B signaling.** *Int Immunopharmacol* 2005, **5**(2):393-406.

129. Meng Y, Ma QY, Kou XP, Xu J: **Effect of resveratrol on activation of nuclear factor kappa-B and inflammatory factors in rat model of acute pancreatitis.** *World J Gastroenterol* 2005, **11**(4):525-528.

130. Juan SH, Cheng TH, Lin HC, Chu YL, Lee WS: **Mechanism of concentration-dependent induction of heme oxygenase-1 by resveratrol in human aortic smooth muscle cells.** *Biochem Pharmacol* 2005, **69**(1):41-48.

131. Kundu JK, Surh YJ: **Molecular basis of chemoprevention by resveratrol: NF-kappaB and AP-1 as potential targets.** *Mutat Res* 2004, **555**(1-2):65-80.

132. Estrov Z, Shishodia S, Faderl S, Harris D, Van Q, Kantarjian HM, Talpaz M, Aggarwal BB: **Resveratrol blocks interleukin-1beta-induced activation of the nuclear transcription factor NF-kappaB, inhibits proliferation, causes S-phase arrest, and induces apoptosis of acute myeloid leukemia cells.** *Blood* 2003, **102**(3):987-995.

133. Adhami VM, Afaq F, Ahmad N: **Suppression of ultraviolet B exposure-mediated activation of NF-kappaB in normal human keratinocytes by resveratrol.** *Neoplasia* 2003, **5**(1):74-82.

134. Ashikawa K, Majumdar S, Banerjee S, Bharti AC, Shishodia S, Aggarwal BB: **Piceatannol inhibits TNF-induced NF-kappaB activation and NF-kappaB-mediated gene expression through suppression of IkappaBalpha kinase and p65 phosphorylation.** *J Immunol* 2002, **169**(11):6490-6497.

135. Manna SK, Mukhopadhyay A, Aggarwal BB: **Resveratrol suppresses TNF-induced activation of nuclear transcription factors NF-kappa B, activator protein-1, and**

apoptosis: potential role of reactive oxygen intermediates and lipid peroxidation. *J Immunol* 2000, **164**(12):6509-6519.

136. Wadsworth TL, Koop DR: **Effects of the wine polyphenolics quercetin and resveratrol on pro-inflammatory cytokine expression in RAW 264.7 macrophages.** *Biochem Pharmacol* 1999, **57**(8):941-949.

137. Woo JH, Lim JH, Kim YH, Suh SI, Min do S, Chang JS, Lee YH, Park JW, Kwon TK: **Resveratrol inhibits phorbol myristate acetate-induced matrix metalloproteinase-9 expression by inhibiting JNK and PKC delta signal transduction.** *Oncogene* 2004, **23**(10):1845-1853.

138. Taubert D, Berkels R: **Upregulation and activation of eNOS by resveratrol.** *Circulation* 2003, **107**(11):e78-79; author reply e78-79.

139. Wallerath T, Deckert G, Ternes T, Anderson H, Li H, Witte K, Forstermann U: **Resveratrol, a polyphenolic phytoalexin present in red wine, enhances expression and activity of endothelial nitric oxide synthase.** *Circulation* 2002, **106**(13):1652-1658.

140. Hsieh TC, Juan G, Darzynkiewicz Z, Wu JM: **Resveratrol increases nitric oxide synthase, induces accumulation of p53 and p21(WAF1/CIP1), and suppresses cultured bovine pulmonary artery endothelial cell proliferation by perturbing progression through S and G2.** *Cancer Res* 1999, **59**(11):2596-2601.

141. Miatello R, Vazquez M, Renna N, Cruzado M, Zumino AP, Risler N: **Chronic administration of resveratrol prevents biochemical cardiovascular changes in fructose-fed rats.** *Am J Hypertens* 2005, **18**(6):864-870.

142. Wallerath T, Li H, Godtel-Ambrust U, Schwarz PM, Forstermann U: **A blend of polyphenolic compounds explains the stimulatory effect of red wine on human endothelial NO synthase.** *Nitric Oxide* 2005, **12**(2):97-104.

143. El-Mowafy AM, White RE: **Resveratrol inhibits MAPK activity and nuclear translocation in coronary artery smooth muscle: reversal of endothelin-1 stimulatory effects.** *FEBS Lett* 1999, **451**(1):63-67.

144. Mizutani K, Ikeda K, Yamori Y: **Resveratrol inhibits AGEs-induced proliferation and collagen synthesis activity in vascular smooth muscle cells from stroke-prone spontaneously hypertensive rats.** *Biochem Biophys Res Commun* 2000, **274**(1):61-67.

145. Zou J, Huang Y, Cao K, Yang G, Yin H, Len J, Hsieh TC, Wu JM: **Effect of resveratrol on intimal hyperplasia after endothelial denudation in an experimental rabbit model.** *Life Sci* 2000, **68**(2):153-163.

146. Araim O, Ballantyne J, Waterhouse AL, Sumpio BE: **Inhibition of vascular smooth muscle cell proliferation with red wine and red wine polyphenols.** *J Vasc Surg* 2002, **35**(6):1226-1232.

147. Chao HH, Juan SH, Liu JC, Yang HY, Yang E, Cheng TH, Shyu KG: **Resveratrol inhibits angiotensin II-induced endothelin-1 gene expression and subsequent proliferation in rat aortic smooth muscle cells.** *Eur J Pharmacol* 2005, **515**(1-3):1-9.

148. Soleas GJ, Diamandis EP, Goldberg DM: **Wine as a biological fluid: history, production, and role in disease prevention.** *J Clin Lab Anal* 1997, **11**(5):287-313.

149. Yamakoshi J, Kataoka S, Koga T, Ariga T: **Proanthocyanidin-rich extract from grape seeds attenuates the development of aortic atherosclerosis in cholesterol-fed rabbits.** *Atherosclerosis* 1999, **142**(1):139-149.

150. Koga T, Moro K, Nakamori K, Yamakoshi J, Hosoyama H, Kataoka S, Ariga T: **Increase of antioxidative potential of rat plasma by oral administration of proanthocyanidin-rich extract from grape seeds.** *J Agric Food Chem* 1999, **47**(5):1892-1897.

151. van de Wiel A, van Golde PH, Hart HC: **Blessings of the grape.** *Eur J Intern Med* 2001, **12**(6):484-489.

152. Deckert V, Desrumaux C, Athias A, Duverneuil L, Palleau V, Gambert P, Masson D, Lagrost L: **Prevention of LDL alpha-tocopherol consumption, cholesterol oxidation, and vascular endothelium dysfunction by polyphenolic compounds from red wine.** *Atherosclerosis* 2002, **165**(1):41-50.

153. van de Wiel A: **[Nutrition and health--favorable effect of wine and wine flavonoids on cardiovascular diseases].** *Ned Tijdschr Geneeskd* 2002, **146**(51):2466-2469.

154. Zern TL, West KL, Fernandez ML: **Grape polyphenols decrease plasma triglycerides and cholesterol accumulation in the aorta of ovariectomized guinea pigs.** *J Nutr* 2003, **133**(7):2268-2272.

155. Miura D, Miura Y, Yagasaki K: **Hypolipidemic action of dietary resveratrol, a phytoalexin in grapes and red wine, in hepatoma-bearing rats.** *Life Sci* 2003, **73**(11):1393-1400.

156. Auger C, Gerain P, Laurent-Bichon F, Portet K, Bornet A, Caporiccio B, Cros G, Teissedre PL, Rouanet JM: **Phenolics from commercialized grape extracts prevent early atherosclerotic lesions in hamsters by mechanisms other than antioxidant effect.** *J Agric Food Chem* 2004, **52**(16):5297-5302.

157. Hansen AS, Marckmann P, Dragsted LO, Finne Nielsen IL, Nielsen SE, Gronbaek M: **Effect of red wine and red grape extract on blood lipids, haemostatic factors, and other risk factors for cardiovascular disease.** *Eur J Clin Nutr* 2005, **59**(3):449-455.

158. de Gaetano G, Di Castelnuovo A, Donati MB, Iacoviello L: **The mediterranean lecture: wine and thrombosis--from epidemiology to physiology and back.** *Pathophysiol Haemost Thromb* 2003, **33**(5-6):466-471.

159. Fuhrman B, Volkova N, Coleman R, Aviram M: **Grape powder polyphenols attenuate atherosclerosis development in apolipoprotein E deficient (E0) mice and reduce macrophage atherogenicity.** *J Nutr* 2005, **135**(4):722-728.

160. Zern TL, Wood RJ, Greene C, West KL, Liu Y, Aggarwal D, Shachter NS, Fernandez ML: **Grape polyphenols exert a cardioprotective effect in pre- and postmenopausal women by lowering plasma lipids and reducing oxidative stress.** *J Nutr* 2005, **135**(8):1911-1917.

161. Del Bas JM, Fernandez-Larrea J, Blay M, Ardevol A, Salvado MJ, Arola L, Blade C: **Grape seed procyanidins improve atherosclerotic risk index and induce liver CYP7A1 and SHP expression in healthy rats.** *Faseb J* 2005, **19**(3):479-481.

162. Gunjima M, Tofani I, Kojima Y, Maki K, Kimura M: **Mechanical evaluation of effect of grape seed proanthocyanidins extract on debilitated mandibles in rats.** *Dent Mater J* 2004, **23**(2):67-74.

163. Mattoo TK, Kovacevic L: **Effect of grape seed extract on puromycin-aminonucleoside-induced nephrosis in rats.** *Pediatr Nephrol* 2003, **18**(9):872-877.

164. Yu H, Zhao X, Xu G, Wang SE: **[Effect of grape seed extracts on blood lipids in rabbits model with hyperlipidemia].** *Wei Sheng Yan Jiu* 2002, **31**(2):114-116.

165. Preuss HG, Montamarry S, Echard B, Scheckenbach R, Bagchi D: **Long-term effects of chromium, grape seed extract, and zinc on various metabolic parameters of rats.** *Mol Cell Biochem* 2001, **223**(1-2):95-102.

166. Shafiee M, Carbonneau MA, Urban N, Descomps B, Leger CL: **Grape and grape seed extract capacities at protecting LDL against oxidation generated by Cu2+, AAPH or SIN-1 and at decreasing superoxide THP-1 cell production. A comparison to other extracts or compounds.** *Free Radic Res* 2003, **37**(5):573-584.

167. Brito P, Almeida LM, Dinis TC: **The interaction of resveratrol with ferrylmyoglobin and peroxynitrite; protection against LDL oxidation.** *Free Radic Res* 2002, **36**(6):621-631.

168. , Young JF, Dragsted LO, Daneshvar B, Lauridsen ST, Hansen M, Sandstrom B: **The effect of grape-skin extract on oxidative status.** *Br J Nutr* 2000, **84**(4):505-513.

169. Berti F, Manfredi B, Mantegazza P, Rossoni G: **Procyanidins from Vitis vinifera seeds display cardioprotection in an experimental model of ischemia-reperfusion damage.** *Drugs Exp Clin Res* 2003, **29**(5-6):207-216.

170. Shao ZH, Becker LB, Vanden Hoek TL, Schumacker PT, Li CQ, Zhao D, Wojcik K, Anderson T, Qin Y, Dey L *et al*: **Grape seed proanthocyanidin extract attenuates oxidant injury in cardiomyocytes.** *Pharmacol Res* 2003, **47**(6):463-469.

171. Sato M, Bagchi D, Tosaki A, Das DK: **Grape seed proanthocyanidin reduces cardiomyocyte apoptosis by inhibiting ischemia/reperfusion-induced activation of JNK-1 and C-JUN.** *Free Radic Biol Med* 2001, **31**(6):729-737.

172. Corder R, Warburton RC, Khan NQ, Brown RE, Wood EG, Lees DM: **The procyanidin-induced pseudo laminar shear stress response: a new concept for the reversal of endothelial dysfunction.** *Clin Sci (Lond)* 2004, **107**(5):513-517.

173. Agarwal C, Singh RP, Dhanalakshmi S, Agarwal R: **Anti-angiogenic efficacy of grape seed extract in endothelial cells.** *Oncol Rep* 2004, **11**(3):681-685.

174. Singh RP, Tyagi AK, Dhanalakshmi S, Agarwal R, Agarwal C: **Grape seed extract inhibits advanced human prostate tumor growth and angiogenesis and upregulates insulin-like growth factor binding protein-3.** *Int J Cancer* 2004, **108**(5):733-740.

175. Aldini G, Carini M, Piccoli A, Rossoni G, Facino RM: **Procyanidins from grape seeds protect endothelial cells from peroxynitrite damage and enhance endothelium-dependent relaxation in human artery: new evidences for cardio-protection.** *Life Sci* 2003, **73**(22):2883-2898.

176. Roy S, Khanna S, Alessio HM, Vider J, Bagchi D, Bagchi M, Sen CK: **Anti-angiogenic property of edible berries.** *Free Radic Res* 2002, **36**(9):1023-1031.

177. Khanna S, Venojarvi M, Roy S, Sharma N, Trikha P, Bagchi D, Bagchi M, Sen CK: **Dermal wound healing properties of redox-active grape seed proanthocyanidins.** *Free Radic Biol Med* 2002, **33**(8):1089-1096.

178. Khanna S, Roy S, Bagchi D, Bagchi M, Sen CK: **Upregulation of oxidant-induced VEGF expression in cultured keratinocytes by a grape seed proanthocyanidin extract.** *Free Radic Biol Med* 2001, **31**(1):38-42.

179. Sen CK, Bagchi D: **Regulation of inducible adhesion molecule expression in human endothelial cells by grape seed proanthocyanidin extract.** *Mol Cell Biochem* 2001, **216**(1-2):1-7.

180. Shao ZH, Vanden Hoek TL, Xie J, Wojcik K, Chan KC, Li CQ, Hamann K, Qin Y, Schumacker PT, Becker LB *et al*: **Grape seed proanthocyanidins induce pro-oxidant toxicity in cardiomyocytes.** *Cardiovasc Toxicol* 2003, **3**(4):331-339.

181. Feng R, He W, Hirotomo O: **[Experimental studies on antioxidation of extracts from several plants used as both medicines and foods in vitro].** *Zhong Yao Cai* 2000, **23**(11):690-693.

182. Roychowdhury S, Wolf G, Keilhoff G, Bagchi D, Horn T: **Protection of primary glial cells by grape seed proanthocyanidin extract against nitrosative/oxidative stress.** *Nitric Oxide* 2001, **5**(2):137-149.

183. Bagchi D, Garg A, Krohn RL, Bagchi M, Bagchi DJ, Balmoori J, Stohs SJ: **Protective effects of grape seed proanthocyanidins and selected antioxidants against TPA-induced hepatic and brain lipid peroxidation and DNA fragmentation, and peritoneal macrophage activation in mice.** *Gen Pharmacol* 1998, **30**(5):771-776.

184. Deshane J, Chaves L, Sarikonda KV, Isbell S, Wilson L, Kirk M, Grubbs C, Barnes S, Meleth S, Kim H: **Proteomics analysis of rat brain protein modulations by grape seed extract.** *J Agric Food Chem* 2004, **52**(26):7872-7883.

185. Johnson-Varghese L, Brodsky N, Bhandari V: **Effect of antioxidants on apoptosis and cytokine release in fetal rat Type II pneumocytes exposed to hyperoxia and nitric oxide.** *Cytokine* 2004, **28**(1):10-16.

186. Kalin R, Righi A, Del Rosso A, Bagchi D, Generini S, Cerinic MM, Das DK: **Activin, a grape seed-derived proanthocyanidin extract, reduces plasma levels of oxidative stress and adhesion molecules (ICAM-1, VCAM-1 and E-selectin) in systemic sclerosis.** *Free Radic Res* 2002, **36**(8):819-825.

187. Li WG, Zhang XY, Wu YJ, Tian X: **Anti-inflammatory effect and mechanism of proanthocyanidins from grape seeds.** *Acta Pharmacol Sin* 2001, **22**(12):1117-1120.

188. Abu-Amsha R, Croft KD, Puddey IB, Proudfoot JM, Beilin LJ: **Phenolic content of various beverages determines the extent of inhibition of human serum and low-density lipoprotein oxidation in vitro: identification and mechanism of action of some cinnamic acid derivatives from red wine.** *Clin Sci (Lond)* 1996, **91**(4):449-458.

189. Puddey IB, Croft KD, Abdu-Amsha Caccetta R, Beilin LJ: **Alcohol, free radicals and antioxidants.** *Novartis Found Symp* 1998, **216**:51-62; discussion 63-57, 152-158.

190. Lee JH, Talcott ST: **Fruit maturity and juice extraction influences ellagic acid derivatives and other antioxidant polyphenolics in muscadine grapes.** *J Agric Food Chem* 2004, **52**(2):361-366.

191. Shi J, Yu J, Pohorly JE, Kakuda Y: **Polyphenolics in grape seeds-biochemistry and functionality.** *J Med Food* 2003, **6**(4):291-299.

192. Pastrana-Bonilla E, Akoh CC, Sellappan S, Krewer G: **Phenolic content and antioxidant capacity of muscadine grapes.** *J Agric Food Chem* 2003, **51**(18):5497-5503.

193. Cantos E, Espin JC, Tomas-Barberan FA: **Varietal differences among the polyphenol profiles of seven table grape cultivars studied by LC-DAD-MS-MS.** *J Agric Food Chem* 2002, **50**(20):5691-5696.

194. Mattivi F, Zulian C, Nicolini G, Valenti L: **Wine, biodiversity, technology, and antioxidants.** *Ann N Y Acad Sci* 2002, **957**:37-56.

195. Young JF, Dragsted LO, Daneshvar B, Lauridsen ST, Hansen M, Sandstrom B: **The effect of grape-skin extract on oxidative status.** *Br J Nutr* 2000, **84**(4):505-513.

196. Blanco VZ, Auw JM, Sims CA, O'Keefe SF: **Effect of processing on phenolics of wines.** *Adv Exp Med Biol* 1998, **434**:327-340.

197. Li MH, Jang JH, Sun B, Surh YJ: **Protective effects of oligomers of grape seed polyphenols against beta-amyloid-induced oxidative cell death.** *Ann N Y Acad Sci* 2004, **1030**:317-329.

198. Vayalil PK, Mittal A, Katiyar SK: **Proanthocyanidins from grape seeds inhibit expression of matrix metalloproteinases in human prostate carcinoma cells, which is associated with the inhibition of activation of MAPK and NF kappa B.** *Carcinogenesis* 2004, **25**(6):987-995.

199. Dhanalakshmi S, Agarwal R, Agarwal C: **Inhibition of NF-kappaB pathway in grape seed extract-induced apoptotic death of human prostate carcinoma DU145 cells.** *Int J Oncol* 2003, **23**(3):721-727.

200. Holmes-McNary M, Baldwin AS, Jr.: **Chemopreventive properties of trans-resveratrol are associated with inhibition of activation of the IkappaB kinase.** *Cancer Res* 2000, **60**(13):3477-3483.

201. Soares De Moura R, Costa Viana FS, Souza MA, Kovary K, Guedes DC, Oliveira EP, Rubenich LM, Carvalho LC, Oliveira RM, Tano T *et al*: **Antihypertensive, vasodilator and antioxidant effects of a vinifera grape skin extract.** *J Pharm Pharmacol* 2002, **54**(11):1515-1520.

202. Burr ML: **Explaining the French paradox.** *J R Soc Health* 1995, **115**(4):217-219.

203. Ulrich S, Wolter F, Stein JM: **Molecular mechanisms of the chemopreventive effects of resveratrol and its analogs in carcinogenesis.** *Mol Nutr Food Res* 2005, **49**(5):452-461.

204. Rasmussen SE, Frederiksen H, Struntze Krogholm K, Poulsen L: **Dietary proanthocyanidins: occurrence, dietary intake, bioavailability, and protection against cardiovascular disease.** *Mol Nutr Food Res* 2005, **49**(2):159-174.

205. Goldfinger TM: **Beyond the French paradox: the impact of moderate beverage alcohol and wine consumption in the prevention of cardiovascular disease.** *Cardiol Clin* 2003, **21**(3):449-457.

206. Brouillard R, Chassaing S, Fougerousse A: **Why are grape/fresh wine anthocyanins so simple and why is it that red wine color lasts so long?** *Phytochemistry* 2003, **64**(7):1179-1186.

207. Petrie JR, Cleland SJ, Small M: **The metabolic syndrome: Overeating, inactivity, poor compliance or 'dud' advice?** *Diabetic Medicine* 1998, **15**(11):S29-S31.

208. Buttriss J, Nugent A: **LIPGENE: an integrated approach to tackling the metabolic syndrome.** *Proc Nutr Soc* 2005, **64**(3):345-347.

209. Nugent AP: **LIPGENE: an EU project to tackle the metabolic syndrome.** *Biochimie* 2005, **87**(1):129-132.

210. Yilmaz Y, Toledo RT: **Major flavonoids in grape seeds and skins: antioxidant capacity of catechin, epicatechin, and gallic acid.** *J Agric Food Chem* 2004, **52**(2):255-260.

211. Zhuang H, Kim YS, Koehler RC, Dore S: **Potential mechanism by which resveratrol, a red wine constituent, protects neurons.** *Ann N Y Acad Sci* 2003, **993**:276-286; discussion 287-278.

212. Jorge AP, Horst H, de Sousa E, Pizzolatti MG, Silva FR: **Insulinomimetic effects of kaempferitrin on glycaemia and on 14C-glucose uptake in rat soleus muscle.** *Chem Biol Interact* 2004, **149**(2-3):89-96.

213. Jung UJ, Lee MK, Jeong KS, Choi MS: **The hypoglycemic effects of hesperidin and naringin are partly mediated by hepatic glucose-regulating enzymes in C57BL/KsJ-db/db mice.** *J Nutr* 2004, **134**(10):2499-2503.

214. Liu X, Wei J, Tan F, Zhou S, Wurthwein G, Rohdewald P: **Antidiabetic effect of Pycnogenol French maritime pine bark extract in patients with diabetes type II.** *Life Sci* 2004, **75**(21):2505-2513.

215. de Sousa E, Zanatta L, Seifriz I, Creczynski-Pasa TB, Pizzolatti MG, Szpoganicz B, Silva FR: **Hypoglycemic effect and antioxidant potential of kaempferol-3,7-O-(alpha)-dirhamnoside from Bauhinia forficata leaves.** *J Nat Prod* 2004, **67**(5):829-832.

216. Anjaneyulu M, Chopra K: **Quercetin, an anti-oxidant bioflavonoid, attenuates diabetic nephropathy in rats.** *Clin Exp Pharmacol Physiol* 2004, **31**(4):244-248.

217. Mahesh T, Menon VP: **Quercetin allievates oxidative stress in streptozotocin-induced diabetic rats.** *Phytother Res* 2004, **18**(2):123-127.

218. Pal S, Naissides M, Mamo J: **Polyphenolics and fat absorption.** *Int J Obes Relat Metab Disord* 2004, **28**(2):324-326.

219. Al-Awwadi N, Azay J, Poucheret P, Cassanas G, Krosniak M, Auger C, Gasc F, Rouanet JM, Cros G, Teissedre PL: **Antidiabetic activity of red wine polyphenolic extract, ethanol, or both in streptozotocin-treated rats.** *J Agric Food Chem* 2004, **52**(4):1008-1016.

220. Martin HJ, Kornmann F, Fuhrmann GF: **The inhibitory effects of flavonoids and antiestrogens on the Glut1 glucose transporter in human erythrocytes.** *Chem Biol Interact* 2003, **146**(3):225-235.

221. Vessal M, Hemmati M, Vasei M: **Antidiabetic effects of quercetin in streptozocin-induced diabetic rats.** *Comp Biochem Physiol C Toxicol Pharmacol* 2003, **135C**(3):357-364.

222. Murota K, Terao J: **Antioxidative flavonoid quercetin: implication of its intestinal absorption and metabolism.** *Arch Biochem Biophys* 2003, **417**(1):12-17.

223. Moharram FA, Marzouk MS, El-Toumy SA, Ahmed AA, Aboutabl EA: **Polyphenols of Melaleuca quinquenervia leaves--pharmacological studies of grandinin.** *Phytother Res* 2003, **17**(7):767-773.

224. Kawanishi K, Ueda H, Moriyasu M: **Aldose reductase inhibitors from the nature.** *Curr Med Chem* 2003, **10**(15):1353-1374.

225. Diebolt M, Bucher B, Andriantsitohaina R: **Wine polyphenols decrease blood pressure, improve NO vasodilatation, and induce gene expression.** *Hypertension* 2001, **38**(2):159-165.

226. Valsa AK, Sudheesh S, Vijayalakshmi NR: **Effect of catechin on carbohydrate metabolism.** *Indian J Biochem Biophys* 1997, **34**(4):406-408.

227. Cignarella A, Nastasi M, Cavalli E, Puglisi L: **Novel lipid-lowering properties of Vaccinium myrtillus L. leaves, a traditional antidiabetic treatment, in several models of rat dyslipidaemia: a comparison with ciprofibrate.** *Thromb Res* 1996, **84**(5):311-322.

228. Varma SD, Richards RD: **Etiology of cataracts in diabetics.** *Int Ophthalmol Clin* 1984, **24**(4):93-110.

229. Varma SD, Schocket SS, Richards RD: **Implications of aldose reductase in cataracts in human diabetes.** *Invest Ophthalmol Vis Sci* 1979, **18**(3):237-241.

230. Clifford MN: **Diet-derived phenols in plasma and tissues and their implications for health.** *Planta Med* 2004, **70**(12):1103-1114.

231. Moreno DA, Ilic N, Poulev A, Brasaemle DL, Fried SK, Raskin I: **Inhibitory effects of grape seed extract on lipases.** *Nutrition* 2003, **19**(10):876-879.

232. Flechtner-Mors M, Biesalski HK, Jenkinson CP, Adler G, Ditschuneit HH: **Effects of moderate consumption of white wine on weight loss in overweight and obese subjects.** *Int J Obes Relat Metab Disord* 2004, **28**(11):1420-1426.

233. Han LK, Sumiyoshi M, Zhang J, Liu MX, Zhang XF, Zheng YN, Okuda H, Kimura Y: **Anti-obesity action of Salix matsudana leaves (Part 1). Anti-obesity action by polyphenols of Salix matsudana in high fat-diet treated rodent animals.** *Phytother Res* 2003, **17**(10):1188-1194.

234. Ector BJ, Dodson WL, Khan FA, Jackson VL: **Effects of muscadine grape supplements on blood lipid of mildly hyperlipemic adults.** *FASEB Journal* 2002, **16**(4):A240.

235. Lunceford N, Gugliucci A: **Ilex paraguariensis extracts inhibit AGE formation more efficiently than green tea.** *Fitoterapia* 2005.

236. Kim HY, Moon BH, Lee HJ, Choi DH: **Flavonol glycosides from the leaves of Eucommia ulmoides O. with glycation inhibitory activity.** *J Ethnopharmacol* 2004, **93**(2-3):227-230.

237. Auger C, Teissedre PL, Gerain P, Lequeux N, Bornet A, Serisier S, Besancon P, Caporiccio B, Cristol JP, Rouanet JM: **Dietary wine phenolics catechin, quercetin, and resveratrol efficiently protect hypercholesterolemic hamsters against aortic fatty streak accumulation.** *J Agric Food Chem* 2005, **53**(6):2015-2021.

238. Al-Awwadi NA, Araiz C, Bornet A, Delbosc S, Cristol JP, Linck N, Azay J, Teissedre PL, Cros G: **Extracts enriched in different polyphenolic families normalize increased cardiac NADPH oxidase expression while having differential effects on insulin resistance, hypertension, and cardiac hypertrophy in high-fructose-fed rats.** *J Agric Food Chem* 2005, **53**(1):151-157.

239. Al-Awwadi NA, Bornet A, Azay J, Araiz C, Delbosc S, Cristol JP, Linck N, Cros G, Teissedre PL: **Red wine polyphenols alone or in association with ethanol prevent hypertension, cardiac hypertrophy, and production of reactive oxygen species in the insulin-resistant fructose-fed rat.** *J Agric Food Chem* 2004, **52**(18):5593-5597.

240. Maron DJ: **Flavonoids for reduction of atherosclerotic risk.** *Curr Atheroscler Rep* 2004, **6**(1):73-78.

241. Zenebe W, Pechanova O: **Effects of red wine polyphenolic compounds on the cardiovascular system.** *Bratisl Lek Listy* 2002, **103**(4-5):159-165.

242. Wang Q, Yu S, Simonyi A, Rottinghaus G, Sun GY, Sun AY: **Resveratrol protects against neurotoxicity induced by kainic acid.** *Neurochem Res* 2004, **29**(11):2105-2112.

243. Yoshikawa M, Shimada H, Nishida N, Li Y, Toguchida I, Yamahara J, Matsuda H: **Antidiabetic principles of natural medicines. II. Aldose reductase and alpha-glucosidase inhibitors from Brazilian natural medicine, the leaves of Myrcia multiflora DC. (Myrtaceae): structures of myrciacitrins I and II and myrciaphenones A and B.** *Chem Pharm Bull (Tokyo)* 1998, **46**(1):113-119.

244. Lim SS, Jung SH, Ji J, Shin KH, Keum SR: **Synthesis of flavonoids and their effects on aldose reductase and sorbitol accumulation in streptozotocin-induced diabetic rat tissues.** *J Pharm Pharmacol* 2001, **53**(5):653-668.

245. Ueda H, Kuroiwa E, Tachibana Y, Kawanishi K, Ayala F, Moriyasu M: **Aldose reductase inhibitors from the leaves of Myrciaria dubia (H. B. & K.) McVaugh.** *Phytomedicine* 2004, **11**(7-8):652-656.

246. Ueda H, Kawanishi K, Moriyasu M: **Effects of ellagic acid and 2-(2,3,6-trihydroxy-4-carboxyphenyl)ellagic acid on sorbitol accumulation in vitro and in vivo.** *Biol Pharm Bull* 2004, **27**(10):1584-1587.

247. Ueda H, Tachibana Y, Moriyasu M, Kawanishi K, Alves SM: **Aldose reductase inhibitors from the fruits of Caesalpinia ferrea Mart.** *Phytomedicine* 2001, **8**(5):377-381.

248. Terashima S, Shimizu M, Horie S, Morita N: **Studies on aldose reductase inhibitors from natural products. IV. Constituents and aldose reductase inhibitory effect of Chrysanthemum morifolium, Bixa orellana and Ipomoea batatas.** *Chem Pharm Bull (Tokyo)* 1991, **39**(12):3346-3347.

249. Terashima S, Shimizu M, Nakayama H, Ishikura M, Ueda Y, Imai K, Suzui A, Morita N: **Studies on aldose reductase inhibitors from medicinal plant of "sinfito," Potentilla candicans, and further synthesis of their related compounds.** *Chem Pharm Bull (Tokyo)* 1990, **38**(10):2733-2736.

250. Shimizu M, Horie S, Terashima S, Ueno H, Hayashi T, Arisawa M, Suzuki S, Yoshizaki M, Morita N: **Studies on aldose reductase inhibitors from natural products. II. Active components of a Paraguayan crude drug "Para-parai mi," Phyllanthus niruri.** *Chem Pharm Bull (Tokyo)* 1989, **37**(9):2531-2532.

251. Haraguchi H, Kanada M, Fukuda A, Naruse K, Okamura N, Yagi A: **An inhibitor of aldose reductase and sorbitol accumulation from Anthocepharus chinensis.** *Planta Med* 1998, **64**(1):68-69.

252. Chaudhry PS, Cabrera J, Juliani HR, Varma SD: **Inhibition of human lens aldose reductase by flavonoids, sulindac and indomethacin.** *Biochem Pharmacol* 1983, **32**(13):1995-1998.

253. Lee Y: **Involvement of nuclear factor kappaB in up-regulation of aldose reductase gene expression by 12-O-tetradecanoylphorbol-13-acetate in HeLa cells.** *Int J Biochem Cell Biol* 2005, **Jun 1.**

254. Manickam M, Ramanathan M, Jahromi MA, Chansouria JP, Ray AB: **Antihyperglycemic activity of phenolics from Pterocarpus marsupium.** *J Nat Prod* 1997, **60**(6):609-610.

255. Landrault N, Poucheret P, Azay J, Krosniak M, Gasc F, Jenin C, Cros G, Teissedre PL: **Effect of a polyphenols-enriched chardonnay white wine in diabetic rats.** *J Agric Food Chem* 2003, **51**(1):311-318.

256. Pinent M, Blay M, Blade MC, Salvado MJ, Arola L, Ardevol A: **Grape seed-derived procyanidins have an antihyperglycemic effect in streptozotocin-induced diabetic rats and insulinomimetic activity in insulin-sensitive cell lines.** *Endocrinology* 2004, **145**(11):4985-4990.

257. Ariga T: **The antioxidative function, preventive action on disease and utilization of proanthocyanidins.** *Biofactors* 2004, **21**(1-4):197-201.

258. El-Alfy AT, Ahmed AA, Fatani AJ: **Protective effect of red grape seeds proanthocyanidins against induction of diabetes by alloxan in rats.** *Pharmacol Res* 2005, **52**(3):264-270.

259. Ong KC, Khoo HE: **Effects of myricetin on glycemia and glycogen metabolism in diabetic rats.** *Life Sci* 2000, **67**(14):1695-1705.

260. Ong KC, Khoo HE: **Insulinomimetic effects of myricetin on lipogenesis and glucose transport in rat adipocytes but not glucose transport translocation.** *Biochem Pharmacol* 1996, **51**(4):423-429.

261. Hemmerle H, Burger HJ, Below P, Schubert G, Rippel R, Schindler PW, Paulus E, Herling AW: **Chlorogenic acid and synthetic chlorogenic acid derivatives: novel inhibitors of hepatic glucose-6-phosphate translocase.** *J Med Chem* 1997, **40**(2):137-145.

262. Rodriguez de Sotillo DV, Hadley M: **Chlorogenic acid modifies plasma and liver concentrations of: cholesterol, triacylglycerol, and minerals in (fa/fa) Zucker rats.** *J Nutr Biochem* 2002, **13**(12):717-726.

263. McCarty MF: **Nutraceutical resources for diabetes prevention--an update.** *Med Hypotheses* 2005, **64**(1):151-158.

264. McCarty MF: **A chlorogenic acid-induced increase in GLP-1 production may mediate the impact of heavy coffee consumption on diabetes risk.** *Med Hypotheses* 2005, **64**(4):848-853.

265. Rizvi SI, Zaid MA, Anis R, Mishra N: **Protective role of tea catechins against oxidation-induced damage of type 2 diabetic erythrocytes.** *Clin Exp Pharmacol Physiol* 2005, **32**(1-2):70-75.

266. Hii CS, Howell SL: **Effects of epicatechin on rat islets of Langerhans.** *Diabetes* 1984, **33**(3):291-296.

267. Chakravarthy BK, Gupta S, Gode KD: **Antidiabetic effect of (-)-epicatechin.** *Lancet* 1982, **2**(8292):272-273.

268. Andrade Cetto A, Wiedenfeld H, Revilla MC, Sergio IA: **Hypoglycemic effect of Equisetum myriochaetum aerial parts on streptozotocin diabetic rats.** *J Ethnopharmacol* 2000, **72**(1-2):129-133.

269. Asgary S, Naderi G, Sarrafzadegan N, Ghassemi N, Boshtam M, Rafie M, Arefian A: **Antioxidant effect of flavonoids on hemoglobin glycosylation.** *Pharm Acta Helv* 1999, **73**(5):223-226.

270. Tsuda T, Horio F, Uchida K, Aoki H, Osawa T: **Dietary cyanidin 3-O-beta-D-glucoside-rich purple corn color prevents obesity and ameliorates hyperglycemia in mice.** *J Nutr* 2003, **133**(7):2125-2130.

271. Tsuda T, Ueno Y, Aoki H, Koda T, Horio F, Takahashi N, Kawada T, Osawa T: **Anthocyanin enhances adipocytokine secretion and adipocyte-specific gene expression in isolated rat adipocytes.** *Biochem Biophys Res Commun* 2004, **316**(1):149-157.

272. Daniel RS, Devi KS, Augusti KT, Sudhakaran Nair CR: **Mechanism of action of antiatherogenic and related effects of Ficus bengalensis Linn. flavonoids in experimental animals.** *Indian J Exp Biol* 2003, **41**(4):296-303.

273. Bertuglia S, Malandrino S, Colantuoni A: **Effects of the natural flavonoid delphinidin on diabetic microangiopathy.** *Arzneimittelforschung* 1995, **45**(4):481-485.

274. Jankowski A, Jankowska B, Niedworok J: [**The effect of anthocyanin dye from grapes on experimental diabetes**]. *Folia Med Cracov* 2000, **41**(3-4):5-15.

275. Matsui T, Ueda T, Oki T, Sugita K, Terahara N, Matsumoto K: **alpha-Glucosidase inhibitory action of natural acylated anthocyanins. 1. Survey of natural pigments with potent inhibitory activity.** *J Agric Food Chem* 2001, **49**(4):1948-1951.

276. Foerster SB, Kizer KW, Disogra LK, Bal DG, Krieg BF, Bunch KL: **California's "5 a day--for better health!" campaign: an innovative population-based effort to effect large-scale dietary change.** *Am J Prev Med* 1995, **11**(2):124-131.

277. Loo G: **Redox-sensitive mechanisms of phytochemical-mediated inhibition of cancer cell proliferation (review).** *J Nutr Biochem* 2003, **14**(2):64-73.

278. Mertens-Talcott SU, Talcott ST, Percival SS: **Low concentrations of quercetin and ellagic acid synergistically influence proliferation, cytotoxicity and apoptosis in MOLT-4 human leukemia cells.** *Journal of Nutrition* 2003, **133**(8):2669-2674.

279. Mertens-Talcott SU, Bomser JA, Talcott ST, Percival SS: **Quercetin and ellagic acid act synergistically in the induction of apoptosis and p21(WAF1/C1P1)-involved signal transduction in human MOLT-4 leukemia cells.** *Faseb Journal* 2004, **18**(4):A379-A379.

280. Mertens-Talcott SU, Bomser JA, Romero C, Talcott ST, Percival SS: **Ellagic acid potentiates the effect of quercetin on p21(wafl/cip1), p53, and MAP-kinases without affecting intracellular generation of reactive oxygen species in vitro.** *Journal of Nutrition* 2005, **135**(3):609-614.

281. Han C, Ding H, Casto B, Stoner GD, D'Ambrosio SM: **Inhibition of the growth of premalignant and malignant human oral cell lines by extracts and components of black raspberries.** *Nutr Cancer* 2005, **51**(2):207-217.

282. Whitley AC, Stoner GD, Darby MV, Walle T: **Intestinal epithelial cell accumulation of the cancer preventive polyphenol ellagic acid--extensive binding to protein and DNA.** *Biochem Pharmacol* 2003, **66**(6):907-915.

283. Narayanan BA, Narayanan NK, Stoner GD, Bullock BP: **Interactive gene expression pattern in prostate cancer cells exposed to phenolic antioxidants.** *Life Sci* 2002, **70**(15):1821-1839.

284. Harris GK, Gupta A, Nines RG, Kresty LA, Habib SG, Frankel WL, LaPerle K, Gallaher DD, Schwartz SJ, Stoner GD: **Effects of lyophilized black raspberries on azoxymethane-induced colon cancer and 8-hydroxy-2'-deoxyguanosine levels in the Fischer 344 rat.** *Nutr Cancer* 2001, **40**(2):125-133.

285. Kresty LA, Morse MA, Morgan C, Carlton PS, Lu J, Gupta A, Blackwood M, Stoner GD: **Chemoprevention of esophageal tumorigenesis by dietary administration of lyophilized black raspberries.** *Cancer Res* 2001, **61**(16):6112-6119.

286. Xue H, Aziz RM, Sun N, Cassady JM, Kamendulis LM, Xu Y, Stoner GD, Klaunig JE: **Inhibition of cellular transformation by berry extracts.** *Carcinogenesis* 2001, **22**(2):351-356.

287. Stoner GD, Kresty LA, Carlton PS, Siglin JC, Morse MA: **Isothiocyanates and freeze-dried strawberries as inhibitors of esophageal cancer.** *Toxicol Sci* 1999, **52**(2 Suppl):95-100.

288. Bohn AA, Forsyth CS, Stoner GD, Reed DJ, Frank AA: **Effect of cocaine, 95% oxygen and ellagic acid on the development and antioxidant status of cultured rat embryos.** *Toxicol Lett* 1998, **95**(1):15-21.

289. Stoner GD, Morse MA: **Isothiocyanates and plant polyphenols as inhibitors of lung and esophageal cancer.** *Cancer Lett* 1997, **114**(1-2):113-119.

290. Harttig U, Hendricks JD, Stoner GD, Bailey GS: **Organ specific, protocol dependent modulation of 7,12-dimethylbenz[a]anthracene carcinogenesis in rainbow trout (Oncorhynchus mykiss) by dietary ellagic acid.** *Carcinogenesis* 1996, **17**(11):2403-2409.

291. Ahn D, Putt D, Kresty L, Stoner GD, Fromm D, Hollenberg PF: **The effects of dietary ellagic acid on rat hepatic and esophageal mucosal cytochromes P450 and phase II enzymes.** *Carcinogenesis* 1996, **17**(4):821-828.

292. Barch DH, Rundhaugen LM, Stoner GD, Pillay NS, Rosche WA: **Structure-function relationships of the dietary anticarcinogen ellagic acid.** *Carcinogenesis* 1996, **17**(2):265-269.

293. Siglin JC, Barch DH, Stoner GD: **Effects of dietary phenethyl isothiocyanate, ellagic acid, sulindac and calcium on the induction and progression of N-nitrosomethylbenzylamine-induced esophageal carcinogenesis in rats.** *Carcinogenesis* 1995, **16**(5):1101-1106.

294. Stoner GD, Mukhtar H: **Polyphenols as cancer chemopreventive agents.** *J Cell Biochem Suppl* 1995, **22**:169-180.

295. Constantinou A, Stoner GD, Mehta R, Rao K, Runyan C, Moon R: **The dietary anticancer agent ellagic acid is a potent inhibitor of DNA topoisomerases in vitro.** *Nutr Cancer* 1995, **23**(2):121-130.

296. Frank AA, Collier JM, Forsyth CS, Zeng W, Stoner GD: **Ellagic acid embryoprotection in vitro: distribution and effects on DNA adduct formation.** *Teratology* 1993, **47**(4):275-280.

297. Stoner GD, Adam-Rodwell G, Morse MA: **Lung tumors in strain A mice: application for studies in cancer chemoprevention.** *J Cell Biochem Suppl* 1993, **17F**:95-103.

298. Heur YH, Zeng W, Stoner GD, Nemeth GA, Hilton B: **Synthesis of ellagic acid O-alkyl derivatives and isolation of ellagic acid as a tetrahexanoyl derivative from Fragaria ananassa.** *J Nat Prod* 1992, **55**(10):1402-1407.

299. Frank AA, Collier JM, Forsyth CS, Heur YH, Stoner GD: **Ellagic acid protects rat embryos in culture from the embryotoxic effects of N-methyl-N-nitrosourea.** *Teratology* 1992, **46**(2):109-115.

300. Daniel EM, Ratnayake S, Kinstle T, Stoner GD: **The effects of pH and rat intestinal contents on the liberation of ellagic acid from purified and crude ellagitannins.** *J Nat Prod* 1991, **54**(4):946-952.

301. Castonguay A, Pepin P, Stoner GD: **Lung tumorigenicity of NNK given orally to A/J mice: its application to chemopreventive efficacy studies.** *Exp Lung Res* 1991, **17**(2):485-499.

302. Daniel EM, Stoner GD: **The effects of ellagic acid and 13-cis-retinoic acid on N-nitrosobenzylmethylamine-induced esophageal tumorigenesis in rats.** *Cancer Lett* 1991, **56**(2):117-124.

303. Mandal S, Stoner GD: **Inhibition of N-nitrosobenzylmethylamine-induced esophageal tumorigenesis in rats by ellagic acid.** *Carcinogenesis* 1990, **11**(1):55-61.

304. Mandal S, Shivapurkar NM, Galati AJ, Stoner GD: **Inhibition of N-nitrosobenzylmethylamine metabolism and DNA binding in cultured rat esophagus by ellagic acid.** *Carcinogenesis* 1988, **9**(7):1313-1316.

305. Mandal S, Ahuja A, Shivapurkar NM, Cheng SJ, Groopman JD, Stoner GD: **Inhibition of aflatoxin B1 mutagenesis in Salmonella typhimurium and DNA damage in cultured rat and human tracheobronchial tissues by ellagic acid.** *Carcinogenesis* 1987, **8**(11):1651-1656.

306. Teel RW, Babcock MS, Dixit R, Stoner GD: **Ellagic acid toxicity and interaction with benzo[a]pyrene and benzo[a]pyrene 7,8-dihydrodiol in human bronchial epithelial cells.** *Cell Biol Toxicol* 1986, **2**(1):53-62.

307. Teel RW, Stoner GD, Babcock MS, Dixit R, Kim K: **Benzo(alpha)pyrene metabolism and DNA-binding in cultured explants of human bronchus and in monolayer cultures of human bronchial epithelial cells treated with ellagic acid.** *Cancer Detect Prev* 1986, **9**(1-2):59-66.

308. Dixit R, Teel RW, Daniel FB, Stoner GD: **Inhibition of benzo(a)pyrene and benzo(a)pyrene-trans-7,8-diol metabolism and DNA binding in mouse lung explants by ellagic acid.** *Cancer Res* 1985, **45**(7):2951-2956.

309. Teel RW, Dixit R, Stoner GD: **The effect of ellagic acid on the uptake, persistence, metabolism and DNA-binding of benzo[a]pyrene in cultured explants of strain A/J mouse lung.** *Carcinogenesis* 1985, **6**(3):391-395.

310. Tate P, God J, Bibb R, Lu Q, Larcom LL: **Inhibition of metalloproteinase activity by fruit extracts.** *Cancer Lett* 2004, **212**(2):153-158.

311. Narayanan BA, Geoffroy O, Willingham MC, Re GG, Nixon DW: **p53/p21(WAF1/CIP1) expression and its possible role in G1 arrest and apoptosis in ellagic acid treated cancer cells.** *Cancer Lett* 1999, **136**(2):215-221.

312. Barch DH, Rundhaugen LM: **Ellagic acid induces NAD(P)H:quinone reductase through activation of the antioxidant responsive element of the rat NAD(P)H:quinone reductase gene.** *Carcinogenesis* 1994, **15**(9):2065-2068.

313. Smart RC, Huang MT, Chang RL, Sayer JM, Jerina DM, Wood AW, Conney AH: **Effect of ellagic acid and 3-O-decylellagic acid on the formation of benzo[a]pyrene-derived DNA adducts in vivo and on the tumorigenicity of 3-methylcholanthrene in mice.** *Carcinogenesis* 1986, **7**(10):1669-1675.

314. Chang RL, Huang MT, Wood AW, Wong CQ, Newmark HL, Yagi H, Sayer JM, Jerina DM, Conney AH: **Effect of ellagic acid and hydroxylated flavonoids on the tumorigenicity of benzo[a]pyrene and (+/-)-7 beta, 8 alpha-dihydroxy-9 alpha, 10 alpha-epoxy-7,8,9,10-tetrahydrobenzo[a]pyrene on mouse skin and in the newborn mouse.** *Carcinogenesis* 1985, **6**(8):1127-1133.

315. Mukhtar H, Das M, Bickers DR: **Inhibition of 3-methylcholanthrene-induced skin tumorigenicity in BALB/c mice by chronic oral feeding of trace amounts of ellagic acid in drinking water.** *Cancer Res* 1986, **46**(5):2262-2265.

316. Mukhtar H, Das M, Del Tito BJ, Jr., Bickers DR: **Protection against 3-methylcholanthrene-induced skin tumorigenesis in Balb/C mice by ellagic acid.** *Biochem Biophys Res Commun* 1984, **119**(2):751-757.

317. Tanaka T, Iwata H, Niwa K, Mori Y, Mori H: **Inhibitory effect of ellagic acid on N-2-fluorenylacetamide-induced liver carcinogenesis in male ACI/N rats.** *Jpn J Cancer Res* 1988, **79**(12):1297-1303.

318. Tanaka T, Kojima T, Kawamori T, Wang A, Suzui M, Okamoto K, Mori H: **Inhibition of 4-nitroquinoline-1-oxide-induced rat tongue carcinogenesis by the naturally occurring plant phenolics caffeic, ellagic, chlorogenic and ferulic acids.** *Carcinogenesis* 1993, **14**(7):1321-1325.

319. Dixit R, Gold B: **Inhibition of N-methyl-N-nitrosourea-induced mutagenicity and DNA methylation by ellagic acid.** *Proc Natl Acad Sci U S A* 1986, **83**(21):8039-8043.

320. Lesca P: **Protective effects of ellagic acid and other plant phenols on benzo[a]pyrene-induced neoplasia in mice.** *Carcinogenesis* 1983, **4**(12):1651-1653.

321. Castonguay A: **Pulmonary carcinogenesis and its prevention by dietary polyphenolic compounds.** *Ann N Y Acad Sci* 1993, **686**:177-185.

322. Barch DH, Fox CC: **Selective inhibition of methylbenzylnitrosamine-induced formation of esophageal O6-methylguanine by dietary ellagic acid in rats.** *Cancer Res* 1988, **48**(24 Pt 1):7088-7092.

323. Krishnan K, Brenner DE: **Chemoprevention of colorectal cancer.** *Gastroenterol Clin North Am* 1996, **25**(4):821-858.

324. Smith WA, Gupta RC: **Use of a microsome-mediated test system to assess efficacy and mechanisms of cancer chemopreventive agents.** *Carcinogenesis* 1996, **17**(6):1285-1290.

325. Barch DH, Fox CC: **Dietary ellagic acid reduces the esophageal microsomal metabolism of methylbenzylnitrosamine.** *Cancer Lett* 1989, **44**(1):39-44.

326. de Boer JG, Yang H, Holcroft J, Skov K: **Chemoprotection against N-nitrosomethylbenzylamine-induced mutation in the rat esophagus.** *Nutr Cancer* 2004, **50**(2):168-173.

327. Maciel ME, Castro GD, Castro JA: **Inhibition of the rat breast cytosolic bioactivation of ethanol to acetaldehyde by some plant polyphenols and folic acid.** *Nutr Cancer* 2004, **49**(1):94-99.

328. Losso JN, Bansode RR, Trappey A, 2nd, Bawadi HA, Truax R: **In vitro anti-proliferative activities of ellagic acid.** *J Nutr Biochem* 2004, **15**(11):672-678.

329. Mertens-Talcott SU, Percival SS: **Ellagic acid and quercetin interact synergistically with resveratrol in the induction of apoptosis and cause transient cell cycle arrest in human leukemia cells.** *Cancer Letters* 2005, **218**(2):141-151.

330. Cerda B, Periago P, Espin JC, Tomas-Barberan FA: **Identification of urolithin a as a metabolite produced by human colon microflora from ellagic acid and related compounds.** *J Agric Food Chem* 2005, **53**(14):5571-5576.

331. Jeong SJ, Kim NY, Kim DH, Kang TH, Ahn NH, Miyamoto T, Higuchi R, Kim YC: **Hyaluronidase inhibitory active 6H-dibenzo[b,d]pyran-6-ones from the feces of Trogopterus xanthipes.** *Planta Med* 2000, **66**(1):76-77.

332. Doyle B, Griffiths LA: **The metabolism of ellagic acid in the rat.** *Xenobiotica* 1980, **10**(4):247-256.

333. Jang M, Cai L, Udeani GO, Slowing KV, Thomas CF, Beecher CW, Fong HH, Farnsworth NR, Kinghorn AD, Mehta RG *et al*: **Cancer chemopreventive activity of resveratrol, a natural product derived from grapes.** *Science* 1997, **275**(5297):218-220.

334. Jang M, Pezzuto JM: **Cancer chemopreventive activity of resveratrol.** *Drugs Exp Clin Res* 1999, **25**(2-3):65-77.

335. Floreani M, Napoli E, Quintieri L, Palatini P: **Oral administration of trans-resveratrol to guinea pigs increases cardiac DT-diaphorase and catalase activities, and protects isolated atria from menadione toxicity.** *Life Sci* 2003, **72**(24):2741-2750.

336. Heo YH, Kim S, Park JE, Jeong LS, Lee SK: **Induction of quinone reductase activity by stilbene analogs in mouse Hepa 1c1c7 cells.** *Arch Pharm Res* 2001, **24**(6):597-600.

337. Aggarwal BB, Bhardwaj A, Aggarwal RS, Seeram NP, Shishodia S, Takada Y: **Role of resveratrol in prevention and therapy of cancer: preclinical and clinical studies.** *Anticancer Res* 2004, **24**(5A):2783-2840.

338. Li YT, Shen F, Liu BH, Cheng GF: **Resveratrol inhibits matrix metalloproteinase-9 transcription in U937 cells.** *Acta Pharmacol Sin* 2003, **24**(11):1167-1171.

339. Oak MH, El Bedoui J, Schini-Kerth VB: **Antiangiogenic properties of natural polyphenols from red wine and green tea.** *J Nutr Biochem* 2005, **16**(1):1-8.

340. Yeung F, Hoberg JE, Ramsey CS, Keller MD, Jones DR, Frye RA, Mayo MW: **Modulation of NF-kappaB-dependent transcription and cell survival by the SIRT1 deacetylase.** *Embo J* 2004, **23**(12):2369-2380.

341. Virgili F, Kobuchi H, Packer L: **Procyanidins extracted from Pinus maritima (Pycnogenol): scavengers of free radical species and modulators of nitrogen monoxide metabolism in activated murine RAW 264.7 macrophages.** *Free Radic Biol Med* 1998, **24**(7-8):1120-1129.

342. Martinez-Florez S, Gutierrez-Fernandez B, Sanchez-Campos S, Gonzalez-Gallego J, Tunon MJ: **Quercetin attenuates nuclear factor-kappaB activation and nitric oxide**

production in interleukin-1beta-activated rat hepatocytes. *J Nutr* 2005, **135**(6):1359-1365.

343. Xu J, Li X, Zhang P, Li ZL, Wang Y: **Antiinflammatory constituents from the roots of Smilax bockii warb.** *Arch Pharm Res* 2005, **28**(4):395-399.

344. Kim AR, Cho JY, Zou Y, Choi JS, Chung HY: **Flavonoids differentially modulate nitric oxide production pathways in lipopolysaccharide-activated RAW264.7 cells.** *Arch Pharm Res* 2005, **28**(3):297-304.

345. Lin R, Liu J, Gan W: **[Protection of vascular endothelial cells from TNF-alpha induced injury by quercetin].** *Zhong Yao Cai* 2004, **27**(8):597-599.

346. Moreira AJ, Fraga C, Alonso M, Collado PS, Zetller C, Marroni C, Marroni N, Gonzalez-Gallego J: **Quercetin prevents oxidative stress and NF-kappaB activation in gastric mucosa of portal hypertensive rats.** *Biochem Pharmacol* 2004, **68**(10):1939-1946.

347. Chen CC, Chow MP, Huang WC, Lin YC, Chang YJ: **Flavonoids inhibit tumor necrosis factor-alpha-induced up-regulation of intercellular adhesion molecule-1 (ICAM-1) in respiratory epithelial cells through activator protein-1 and nuclear factor-kappaB: structure-activity relationships.** *Mol Pharmacol* 2004, **66**(3):683-693.

348. Cho SY, Park SJ, Kwon MJ, Jeong TS, Bok SH, Choi WY, Jeong WI, Ryu SY, Do SH, Lee CS *et al*: **Quercetin suppresses proinflammatory cytokines production through MAP kinases andNF-kappaB pathway in lipopolysaccharide-stimulated macrophage.** *Mol Cell Biochem* 2003, **243**(1-2):153-160.

349. Mu MM, Chakravortty D, Sugiyama T, Koide N, Takahashi K, Mori I, Yoshida T, Yokochi T: **The inhibitory action of quercetin on lipopolysaccharide-induced nitric oxide production in RAW 264.7 macrophage cells.** *J Endotoxin Res* 2001, **7**(6):431-438.

350. Hou DX, Fujii M, Terahara N, Yoshimoto M: **Molecular Mechanisms Behind the Chemopreventive Effects of Anthocyanidins.** *J Biomed Biotechnol* 2004, **2004**(5):321-325.

351. Afaq F, Saleem M, Krueger CG, Reed JD, Mukhtar H: **Anthocyanin- and hydrolyzable tannin-rich pomegranate fruit extract modulates MAPK and NF-kappaB pathways and inhibits skin tumorigenesis in CD-1 mice.** *Int J Cancer* 2005, **113**(3):423-433.

352. Nardini M, Leonardi F, Scaccini C, Virgili F: **Modulation of ceramide-induced NF-kappaB binding activity and apoptotic response by caffeic acid in U937 cells: comparison with other antioxidants.** *Free Radic Biol Med* 2001, **30**(7):722-733.

353. Marquez N, Sancho R, Macho A, Calzado MA, Fiebich BL, Munoz E: **Caffeic acid phenethyl ester inhibits T-cell activation by targeting both nuclear factor of activated T-cells and NF-kappaB transcription factors.** *J Pharmacol Exp Ther* 2004, **308**(3):993-1001.

354. Lin MW, Yang SR, Huang MH, Wu SN: **Stimulatory actions of caffeic acid phenethyl ester, a known inhibitor of NF-kappaB activation, on Ca2+-activated K+ current in pituitary GH3 cells.** *J Biol Chem* 2004, **279**(26):26885-26892.

355. Wang SY, Feng R, Bowman L, Penhallegon R, Ding M, Lu Y: **Antioxidant activity in lingonberries (Vaccinium vitis-idaea L.) and its inhibitory effect on activator protein-1, nuclear factor-kappaB, and mitogen-activated protein kinases activation.** *J Agric Food Chem* 2005, **53**(8):3156-3166.

356. Mousa SS, Mousa SA: **Effect of resveratrol on angiogenesis and platelet/fibrin-accelerated tumor growth in the chick chorioallantoic membrane model.** *Nutr Cancer* 2005, **52**(1):59-65.

357. Azios NG, Dharmawardhane SF: **Resveratrol and estradiol exert disparate effects on cell migration, cell surface actin structures, and focal adhesion assembly in MDA-MB-231 human breast cancer cells.** *Neoplasia* 2005, **7**(2):128-140.

358. Dulak J: **Nutraceuticals as anti-angiogenic agents: hopes and reality.** *J Physiol Pharmacol* 2005, **56 Suppl 1**:51-69.

359. Belleri M, Ribatti D, Nicoli S, Cotelli F, Forti L, Vannini V, Stivala LA, Presta M: **Antiangiogenic and vascular-targeting activity of the microtubule-destabilizing trans-resveratrol derivative 3,5,4'-trimethoxystilbene.** *Mol Pharmacol* 2005, **67**(5):1451-1459.

360. Aggarwal BB, Takada Y, Oommen OV: **From chemoprevention to chemotherapy: common targets and common goals.** *Expert Opin Investig Drugs* 2004, **13**(10):1327-1338.

361. Cao Z, Fang J, Xia C, Shi X, Jiang BH: **trans-3,4,5'-Trihydroxystibene inhibits hypoxia-inducible factor 1alpha and vascular endothelial growth factor expression in human ovarian cancer cells.** *Clin Cancer Res* 2004, **10**(15):5253-5263.

362. Tseng SH, Lin SM, Chen JC, Su YH, Huang HY, Chen CK, Lin PY, Chen Y: **Resveratrol suppresses the angiogenesis and tumor growth of gliomas in rats.** *Clin Cancer Res* 2004, **10**(6):2190-2202.

363. Bianchini F, Vainio H: **Wine and resveratrol: mechanisms of cancer prevention?** *Eur J Cancer Prev* 2003, **12**(5):417-425.

364. Cao Y, Cao R, Brakenhielm E: **Antiangiogenic mechanisms of diet-derived polyphenols.** *J Nutr Biochem* 2002, **13**(7):380-390.

365. Igura K, Ohta T, Kuroda Y, Kaji K: **Resveratrol and quercetin inhibit angiogenesis in vitro.** *Cancer Lett* 2001, **171**(1):11-16.

366. Brakenhielm E, Cao R, Cao Y: **Suppression of angiogenesis, tumor growth, and wound healing by resveratrol, a natural compound in red wine and grapes.** *Faseb J* 2001, **15**(10):1798-1800.

367. Labrecque L, Lamy S, Chapus A, Mihoubi S, Durocher Y, Cass B, Bojanowski MW, Gingras D, Beliveau R: **Combined inhibition of PDGF and VEGF receptors by ellagic acid, a dietary-derived phenolic compound.** *Carcinogenesis* 2005, **26**(4):821-826.

368. Kanadaswami C, Lee LT, Lee PP, Hwang JJ, Ke FC, Huang YT, Lee MT: **The antitumor activities of flavonoids.** *In Vivo* 2005, **19**(5):895-909.

369. Ren W, Qiao Z, Wang H, Zhu L, Zhang L: **Flavonoids: promising anticancer agents.** *Med Res Rev* 2003, **23**(4):519-534.

370. Hollman PC, Katan MB: **Health effects and bioavailability of dietary flavonols.** *Free Radic Res* 1999, **31 Suppl**:S75-80.

371. Williamson G, Manach C: **Bioavailability and bioefficacy of polyphenols in humans. II. Review of 93 intervention studies.** *Am J Clin Nutr* 2005, **81**(1 Suppl):243S-255S.

372. Sampson L, Rimm E, Hollman PC, de Vries JH, Katan MB: **Flavonol and flavone intakes in US health professionals.** *J Am Diet Assoc* 2002, **102**(10):1414-1420.

373. Hollman PC, Bijsman MN, van Gameren Y, Cnossen EP, de Vries JH, Katan MB: **The sugar moiety is a major determinant of the absorption of dietary flavonoid glycosides in man.** *Free Radic Res* 1999, **31**(6):569-573.

374. Arts IC, Sesink AL, Faassen-Peters M, Hollman PC: **The type of sugar moiety is a major determinant of the small intestinal uptake and subsequent biliary excretion of dietary quercetin glycosides.** *Br J Nutr* 2004, **91**(6):841-847.

375. Rechner AR, Kuhnle G, Bremner P, Hubbard GP, Moore KP, Rice-Evans CA: **The metabolic fate of dietary polyphenols in humans.** *Free Radic Biol Med* 2002, **33**(2):220-235.

376. Spencer JP, Kuhnle GG, Williams RJ, Rice-Evans C: **Intracellular metabolism and bioactivity of quercetin and its in vivo metabolites.** *Biochem J* 2003, **372**(Pt 1):173-181.

377. Manach C, Williamson G, Morand C, Scalbert A, Remesy C: **Bioavailability and bioefficacy of polyphenols in humans. I. Review of 97 bioavailability studies.** *Am J Clin Nutr* 2005, **81**(1 Suppl):230S-242S.

378. Mertens SU, Talcott ST, Percival SS: **Low concentrations of quercetin and ellagic acid influence proliferation, cytotoxity and apoptosis in MOLT-4 human leukemic cell in a synergistic manner.** *FASEB Journal* 2003, **17**(4-5):Abstract No. 693.693.

379. Mertens SU, Percival SS: **Low concentrations of polyphenol combinations from red muscadine grapes markedly influence cell cycle kinetics and viability in MOLT-4 cells.** *Faseb Journal* 2002, **16**(5):A1003-A1003.

380. Larrosa M, Tomas-Barberan FA, Espin JC: **The grape and wine polyphenol piceatannol is a potent inducer of apoptosis in human SK-Mel-28 melanoma cells.** *Eur J Nutr* 2004, **43**(5):275-284.

381. Larrosa M, Tomas-Barberan FA, Espin JC: **Grape polyphenol resveratrol and the related molecule 4-hydroxystilbene induce growth inhibition, apoptosis, S-phase**

arrest, and upregulation of cyclins **A, E, and B1 in human SK-Mel-28 melanoma cells.** *J Agric Food Chem* 2003, **51**(16):4576-4584.

382. Cantos E, Espin JC, Fernandez MJ, Oliva J, Tomas-Barberan FA: **Postharvest UV-C-irradiated grapes as a potential source for producing stilbene-enriched red wines.** *J Agric Food Chem* 2003, **51**(5):1208-1214.

383. Cantos E, Espin JC, Tomas-Barberan FA: **Postharvest stilbene-enrichment of red and white table grape varieties using UV-C irradiation pulses.** *J Agric Food Chem* 2002, **50**(22):6322-6329.

384. Gill MT, Bajaj R, Chang CJ, Nichols DE, McLaughlin JL: **3,3',5'-Tri-O-methylpiceatannol and 4,3',5'-tri-O-methylpiceatannol: improvements over piceatannol in bioactivity.** *J Nat Prod* 1987, **50**(1):36-40.

385. Wolter F, Clausnitzer A, Akoglu B, Stein J: **Piceatannol, a natural analog of resveratrol, inhibits progression through the S phase of the cell cycle in colorectal cancer cell lines.** *J Nutr* 2002, **132**(2):298-302.

386. Waffo-Teguo P, Hawthorne ME, Cuendet M, Merillon JM, Kinghorn AD, Pezzuto JM, Mehta RG: **Potential cancer-chemopreventive activities of wine stilbenoids and flavans extracted from grape (Vitis vinifera) cell cultures.** *Nutr Cancer* 2001, **40**(2):173-179.

387. Yang GX, Zhou JT, Li YZ, Hu CQ: **Anti-HIV bioactive stilbene dimers of Caragana rosea.** *Planta Med* 2005, **71**(6):569-571.

388. Vitrac X, Bornet A, Vanderlinde R, Valls J, Richard T, Delaunay JC, Merillon JM, Teissedre PL: **Determination of stilbenes (delta-viniferin, trans-astringin, trans-piceid, cis- and trans-resveratrol, epsilon-viniferin) in Brazilian wines.** *J Agric Food Chem* 2005, **53**(14):5664-5669.

389. Merillon JM, Fauconneau B, Teguo PW, Barrier L, Vercauteren J, Huguet F: **Antioxidant activity of the stilbene astringin, newly extracted from Vitis vinifera cell cultures.** *Clin Chem* 1997, **43**(6 Pt 1):1092-1093.

390. Hougee S, Faber J, Sanders A, de Jong RB, van den Berg WB, Garssen J, Hoijer MA, Smit HF: **Selective COX-2 inhibition by a Pterocarpus marsupium extract characterized by pterostilbene, and its activity in healthy human volunteers.** *Planta Med* 2005, **71**(5):387-392.

391. Tolomeo M, Grimaudo S, Di Cristina A, Roberti M, Pizzirani D, Meli M, Dusonchet L, Gebbia N, Abbadessa V, Crosta L *et al*: **Pterostilbene and 3'-hydroxypterostilbene are effective apoptosis-inducing agents in MDR and BCR-ABL-expressing leukemia cells.** *Int J Biochem Cell Biol* 2005, **37**(8):1709-1726.

392. Ferrer P, Asensi M, Segarra R, Ortega A, Benlloch M, Obrador E, Varea MT, Asensio G, Jorda L, Estrela JM: **Association between pterostilbene and quercetin inhibits metastatic activity of B16 melanoma.** *Neoplasia* 2005, **7**(1):37-47.

393. Rimando AM, Cuendet M, Desmarchelier C, Mehta RG, Pezzuto JM, Duke SO: **Cancer chemopreventive and antioxidant activities of pterostilbene, a naturally occurring analogue of resveratrol.** *J Agric Food Chem* 2002, **50**(12):3453-3457.

394. Lee JY, Kim JH, Kang SS, Bae CS, Choi SH: **The effects of alpha-viniferin on adjuvant-induced arthritis in rats.** *Am J Chin Med* 2004, **32**(4):521-530.

395. Szewczuk LM, Lee SH, Blair IA, Penning TM: **Viniferin formation by COX-1: evidence for radical intermediates during co-oxidation of resveratrol.** *J Nat Prod* 2005, **68**(1):36-42.

396. Quiney C, Dauzonne D, Kern C, Fourneron JD, Izard JC, Mohammad RM, Kolb JP, Billard C: **Flavones and polyphenols inhibit the NO pathway during apoptosis of leukemia B-cells.** *Leuk Res* 2004, **28**(8):851-861.

397. Kang JH, Park YH, Choi SW, Yang EK, Lee WJ: **Resveratrol derivatives potently induce apoptosis in human promyelocytic leukemia cells.** *Exp Mol Med* 2003, **35**(6):467-474.

398. Chung EY, Kim BH, Lee MK, Yun YP, Lee SH, Min KR, Kim Y: **Anti-inflammatory effect of the oligomeric stilbene alpha-Viniferin and its mode of the action through

inhibition of cyclooxygenase-2 and inducible nitric oxide synthase. *Planta Med* 2003, **69**(8):710-714.

399. Billard C, Izard JC, Roman V, Kern C, Mathiot C, Mentz F, Kolb JP: **Comparative antiproliferative and apoptotic effects of resveratrol, epsilon-viniferin and vine-shots derived polyphenols (vineatrols) on chronic B lymphocytic leukemia cells and normal human lymphocytes.** *Leuk Lymphoma* 2002, **43**(10):1991-2002.

400. Lee SH, Shin NH, Kang SH, Park JS, Chung SR, Min KR, Kim Y: **Alpha-viniferin: a prostaglandin H2 synthase inhibitor from root of Carex humilis.** *Planta Med* 1998, **64**(3):204-207.

401. Kitanaka S, Ikezawa T, Yasukawa K, Yamanouchi S, Takido M, Sung HK, Kim IH: **(+)-Alpha-viniferin, an anti-inflammatory compound from Caragana chamlagu root.** *Chem Pharm Bull (Tokyo)* 1990, **38**(2):432-435.

402. Xu G, Zhang LP, Chen LF, Hu CQ: **[Inhibition of protein kinase C by stilbenoids].** *Yao Xue Xue Bao* 1994, **29**(11):818-822.

403. Regev-Shoshani G, Shoseyov O, Kerem Z: **Influence of lipophilicity on the interactions of hydroxy stilbenes with cytochrome P450 3A4.** *Biochem Biophys Res Commun* 2004, **323**(2):668-673.

404. Moreno-Labanda JF, Mallavia R, Perez-Fons L, Lizama V, Saura D, Micol V: **Determination of piceid and resveratrol in Spanish wines deriving from Monastrell (Vitis vinifera L.) grape variety.** *J Agric Food Chem* 2004, **52**(17):5396-5403.

405. Henry C, Vitrac X, Decendit A, Ennamany R, Krisa S, Merillon JM: **Cellular uptake and efflux of trans-piceid and its aglycone trans-resveratrol on the apical membrane of human intestinal Caco-2 cells.** *J Agric Food Chem* 2005, **53**(3):798-803.

406. Romero-Perez AI, Lamuela-Raventos RM, Andres-Lacueva C, de La Torre-Boronat MC: **Method for the quantitative extraction of resveratrol and piceid isomers in grape berry skins. Effect of powdery mildew on the stilbene content.** *J Agric Food Chem* 2001, **49**(1):210-215.

407. Kimura Y, Okuda H: **Effects of naturally occurring stilbene glucosides from medicinal plants and wine, on tumour growth and lung metastasis in Lewis lung carcinoma-bearing mice.** *J Pharm Pharmacol* 2000, **52**(10):1287-1295.

408. Seeram NP, Adams LS, Hardy ML, Heber D: **Total cranberry extract versus its phytochemical constituents: antiproliferative and synergistic effects against human tumor cell lines.** *J Agric Food Chem* 2004, **52**(9):2512-2517.

409. Zhao J, Wang J, Chen Y, Agarwal R: **Anti-tumor-promoting activity of a polyphenolic fraction isolated from grape seeds in the mouse skin two-stage initiation-promotion protocol and identification of procyanidin B5-3'-gallate as the most effective antioxidant constituent.** *Carcinogenesis* 1999, **20**(9):1737-1745.

410. Jung KJ, Wallig MA, Singletary KW: **Purple grape juice inhibits 7,12-dimethylbenz[a]anthracene (DMBA)-induced rat mammary tumorigenesis and in vivo DMBA-DNA adduct formation.** *Cancer Lett* 2005.

411. Zhang Y, Vareed SK, Nair MG: **Human tumor cell growth inhibition by nontoxic anthocyanidins, the pigments in fruits and vegetables.** *Life Sci* 2005, **76**(13):1465-1472.

412. Singletary KW, Stansbury MJ, Giusti M, Van Breemen RB, Wallig M, Rimando A: **Inhibition of rat mammary tumorigenesis by concord grape juice constituents.** *J Agric Food Chem* 2003, **51**(25):7280-7286.

413. Bagchi D, Sen CK, Bagchi M, Atalay M: **Anti-angiogenic, antioxidant, and anti-carcinogenic properties of a novel anthocyanin-rich berry extract formula.** *Biochemistry (Mosc)* 2004, **69**(1):75-80, 71 p preceding 75.

414. Meiers S, Kemeny M, Weyand U, Gastpar R, von Angerer E, Marko D: **The anthocyanidins cyanidin and delphinidin are potent inhibitors of the epidermal growth-factor receptor.** *J Agric Food Chem* 2001, **49**(2):958-962.

415. Joshi SS, Kuszynski CA, Bagchi M, Bagchi D: **Chemopreventive effects of grape seed proanthocyanidin extract on Chang liver cells.** *Toxicology* 2000, **155**(1-3):83-90.

416. Agarwal C, Singh RP, Agarwal R: **Grape seed extract induces apoptotic death of human prostate carcinoma DU145 cells via caspases activation accompanied by**

dissipation of mitochondrial membrane potential and cytochrome c release. *Carcinogenesis* 2002, **23**(11):1869-1876.

417. Agarwal C, Sharma Y, Agarwal R: **Anticarcinogenic effect of a polyphenolic fraction isolated from grape seeds in human prostate carcinoma DU145 cells: modulation of mitogenic signaling and cell-cycle regulators and induction of G1 arrest and apoptosis.** *Mol Carcinog* 2000, **28**(3):129-138.

418. Engeli S, Schling P, Gorzelniak K, Boschmann M, Janke J, Ailhaud G, Teboul M, Massiera F, Sharma AM: **The adipose-tissue renin-angiotensin-aldosterone system: role in the metabolic syndrome?** *Int J Biochem Cell Biol* 2003, **35**(6):807-825.

419. Carroll S, Dudfield M: **What is the relationship between exercise and metabolic abnormalities? A review of the metabolic syndrome.** *Sports Med* 2004, **34**(6):371-418.

420. Freedland ES: **Role of a critical visceral adipose tissue threshold (CVATT) in metabolic syndrome: implications for controlling dietary carbohydrates: a review.** *Nutr Metab (Lond)* 2004, **1**(1):12.

421. Ridker PM: **C-reactive protein in 2005. Interview by Peter C. Block.** *J Am Coll Cardiol* 2005, **46**(1):CS2-5.

422. Patrick L, Uzick M: **Cardiovascular disease: C-reactive protein and the inflammatory disease paradigm: HMG-CoA reductase inhibitors, alpha-tocopherol, red yeast rice, and olive oil polyphenols. A review of the literature.** *Altern Med Rev* 2001, **6**(3):248-271.

423. de Ferranti S, Rifai N: **C-reactive protein and cardiovascular disease: a review of risk prediction and interventions.** *Clin Chim Acta* 2002, **317**(1-2):1-15.

424. Yeh ET: **CRP as a mediator of disease.** *Circulation* 2004, **109**(21 Suppl 1):II11-14.

425. Yeh ET: **C-reactive protein is an essential aspect of cardiovascular risk factor stratification.** *Can J Cardiol* 2004, **20**(Suppl B):93B-96B.

426. Verma S, Yeh ET: **C-reactive protein and atherothrombosis--beyond a biomarker: an actual partaker of lesion formation.** *Am J Physiol Regul Integr Comp Physiol* 2003, **285**(5):R1253-1256; discussion R1257-1258.

427. Yeh ET, Palusinski RP: **C-reactive protein: the pawn has been promoted to queen.** *Curr Atheroscler Rep* 2003, **5**(2):101-105.

428. Yeh ET, Willerson JT: **Coming of age of C-reactive protein: using inflammation markers in cardiology.** *Circulation* 2003, **107**(3):370-371.

429. Yeh ET, Anderson HV, Pasceri V, Willerson JT: **C-reactive protein: linking inflammation to cardiovascular complications.** *Circulation* 2001, **104**(9):974-975.

430. Greenspan P, Bauer JD, Pollock SH, Hargrove JL, Hartle DK: **Anti-inflammatory properties of the muscadine grape.** *FASEB Journal* 2004, **18**(4-5):Abst. 102.106.

431. Fragopoulou E, Antonopoulou S, Demopoulos CA: **Biologically active lipids with antiatherogenic properties from white wine and must.** *J Agric Food Chem* 2002, **50**(9):2684-2694.

432. Fragopoulou E, Nomikos T, Tsantila N, Mitropoulou A, Zabetakis I, Demopoulos CA: **Biological activity of total lipids from red and white wine/must.** *J Agric Food Chem* 2001, **49**(11):5186-5193.

433. Fragopoulou E, Nomikos T, Antonopoulou S, Mitsopoulou CA, Demopoulos CA: **Separation of biologically active lipids from red wine.** *J Agric Food Chem* 2000, **48**(4):1234-1238.

434. Fragopoulou E, Antonopoulou S, Nomikos T, Demopoulos CA: **Structure elucidation of phenolic compounds from red/white wine with antiatherogenic properties.** *Biochim Biophys Acta* 2003, **1632**(1-3):90-99.

435. Chang WC, Hsu FL: **Inhibition of platelet aggregation and arachidonate metabolism in platelets by procyanidins.** *Prostaglandins Leukot Essent Fatty Acids* 1989, **38**(3):181-188.

436. Winn DM: **Diet and nutrition in the etiology of oral cancer.** *Am J Clin Nutr* 1995, **61**(2):437S-445S.

437. Connolly GN, Winn DM, Hecht SS, Henningfield JE, Walker B, Jr., Hoffmann D: **The reemergence of smokeless tobacco.** *N Engl J Med* 1986, **314**(16):1020-1027.

438. Elattar TM, Virji AS: **The effect of red wine and its components on growth and proliferation of human oral squamous carcinoma cells.** *Anticancer Res* 1999, **19**(6B):5407-5414.

439. Seeram NP, Adams LS, Henning SM, Niu Y, Zhang Y, Nair MG, Heber D: **In vitro antiproliferative, apoptotic and antioxidant activities of punicalagin, ellagic acid and a total pomegranate tannin extract are enhanced in combination with other polyphenols as found in pomegranate juice.** *J Nutr Biochem* 2005, **16**(6):360-367.

440. Aziz MH, Kumar R, Ahmad N: **Cancer chemoprevention by resveratrol: in vitro and in vivo studies and the underlying mechanisms (review).** *Int J Oncol* 2003, **23**(1):17-28.

441. Lambert JD, Hong J, Yang GY, Liao J, Yang CS: **Inhibition of carcinogenesis by polyphenols: evidence from laboratory investigations.** *Am J Clin Nutr* 2005, **81**(1 Suppl):284S-291S.

442. Shirataki Y, Kawase M, Saito S, Kurihara T, Tanaka W, Satoh K, Sakagami H, Motohashi N: **Selective cytotoxic activity of grape peel and seed extracts against oral tumor cell lines.** *Anticancer Res* 2000, **20**(1A):423-426.

443. Thomas G, Hashibe M, Jacob BJ, Ramadas K, Mathew B, Sankaranarayanan R, Zhang ZF: **Risk factors for multiple oral premalignant lesions.** *Int J Cancer* 2003, **107**(2):285-291.

444. McLaughlin JK, Gridley G, Block G, Winn DM, Preston-Martin S, Schoenberg JB, Greenberg RS, Stemhagen A, Austin DF, Ershow AG *et al*: **Dietary factors in oral and pharyngeal cancer.** *J Natl Cancer Inst* 1988, **80**(15):1237-1243.

445. Iwasaki Y, Matsui T, Arakawa Y: **The protective and hormonal effects of proanthocyanidin against gastric mucosal injury in Wistar rats.** *J Gastroenterol* 2004, **39**(9):831-837.

446. Kanner J, Lapidot T: **The stomach as a bioreactor: dietary lipid peroxidation in the gastric fluid and the effects of plant-derived antioxidants.** *Free Radic Biol Med* 2001, **31**(11):1388-1395.

447. Halliwell B, Rafter J, Jenner A: **Health promotion by flavonoids, tocopherols, tocotrienols, and other phenols: direct or indirect effects? Antioxidant or not?** *Am J Clin Nutr* 2005, **81**(1 Suppl):268S-276S.

448. Bao Y, Fenwick R: **Phytochemicals in Health and Disease**. New York: Marcel Dekker; 2004.

449. Johnson MK, Loo G: **Effects of epigallocatechin gallate and quercetin on oxidative damage to cellular DNA.** *Mutat Res* 2000, **459**(3):211-218.

450. Johnson IT: **New food components and gastrointestinal health.** *Proc Nutr Soc* 2001, **60**(4):481-488.

451. Gee JM, Johnson IT: **Polyphenolic compounds: interactions with the gut and implications for human health.** *Curr Med Chem* 2001, **8**(11):1245-1255.

452. Bruch J: **Determining the influence that muscadine fiber has on the production of butyric acid in the rat cecum.** *MS*. Jackson: Mississippi State; 1998.

453. Spiller GA, Story JA, Furumoto EJ, Chezem JC, Spiller M: **Effect of tartaric acid and dietary fibre from sun-dried raisins on colonic function and on bile acid and volatile fatty acid excretion in healthy adults.** *Br J Nutr* 2003, **90**(4):803-807.

454. Spiller GA, Story JA, Lodics TA, Pollack M, Monyan S, Butterfield G, Spiller M: **Effect of sun-dried raisins on bile acid excretion, intestinal transit time, and fecal weight: a dose-response study.** *J Med Food* 2003, **6**(2):87-91.

455. Hertog MG, Bueno-de-Mesquita HB, Fehily AM, Sweetnam PM, Elwood PC, Kromhout D: **Fruit and vegetable consumption and cancer mortality in the Caerphilly Study.** *Cancer Epidemiol Biomarkers Prev* 1996, **5**(9):673-677.

456. Fraser GE, Shavlik DJ: **Ten years of life: Is it a matter of choice?** *Arch Intern Med* 2001, **161**(13):1645-1652.

457. Sinclair DA: **Toward a unified theory of caloric restriction and longevity regulation.** *Mech Ageing Dev* 2005, **126**(9):987-1002.

458. Bordone L, Guarente L: **Calorie restriction, SIRT1 and metabolism: understanding longevity.** *Nat Rev Mol Cell Biol* 2005, **6**(4):298-305.